KETTLEBELL KICKBOXING

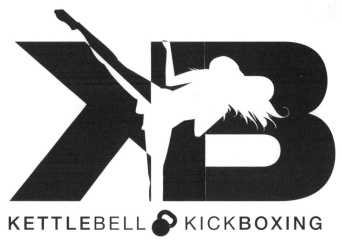

KETTLEBELL KICKBOXING

Every Woman's Guide to Getting Healthy, Sexy, and Strong

by Dasha Libin Anderson

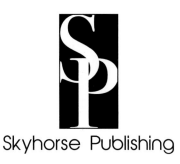

Skyhorse Publishing

Visit our website at www.skyhorsepublishing.com.

10 9 8 7 6 5 4 3 2 1

Library of Congress Cataloging-in-Publication Data is available on file.

Cover design by Rain Saukas
Front cover and chapter introduction photos by Amy Jackson
Back cover and step-by-step photos by Natanya Mitchell of B. Mitchell Studios
Front cover photo and photo on page 7, Shutterstock/Deymos.HR
Photo on page 15, Shutterstock/d9000
Photo model credits: Blue Jung and Jenel Stevens

Print ISBN: 978-1-63220-502-5
Ebook ISBN: 978-1-63220-870-5

Printed in China

Disclaimer
The fitness and nutritional information in this book is meant to supplement, not replace, the advice of a medical, nutritional, and/or fitness professional. Neither the author nor the publisher takes any responsibility for any injury, pain, or other damage related to the use or misuse of this book. It is the responsibility of the reader to be mindful of his or her safety and to know his or her limits. Do not take risks beyond your level of experience, aptitude, training, and comfort.

As with any bodybuilding, exercise, fitness, health, or nutrition book, we strongly advise that you get the approval of a qualified medical/health authority before beginning any exercise program or making any dietary changes. The authors, publisher, people featured, or anyone associated with this book in any way shall not be held liable for anyone's actions either directly or indirectly.

DEDICATION

First and foremost, I dedicate this book to my family. We are not the largest in numbers, but boy, are we strong when we stand together.

To my husband, without whom none of my milestones would be possible: you are my counterpart, my best friend, someone I look up to daily, and I love you.

I would not be who I am today without the strong women who raised me and led by example in their own lives. My mother is my greatest source of inspiration, followed only by my sister, my grandmother, and my niece. Bella, you are my family too.

Jenel, Blue, and Natanya, I asked and you came and helped me put this book together. You are true friends and women of constant inspiration. I look up to each of you, and I thank you.

Jenny, my editor, you found KB and you foresaw this as a book. Thank you for having that vision.

Lastly, and mainly, I dedicated this book to all of the Kettlebell Kickboxers in my classes and around the world! Those of you sweating with me at home and those I see daily, you are my constant motivation, and this book belongs as much to you as it does to me. Thank you for trusting me with your goals and your bodies. You inspire me, and I value all of you deeply. Now go on and get sweaty!

TABLE OF CONTENTS

MY STORY AND AN INTRODUCTION TO THE KETTLEBELL KICKBOXING PROGRAM

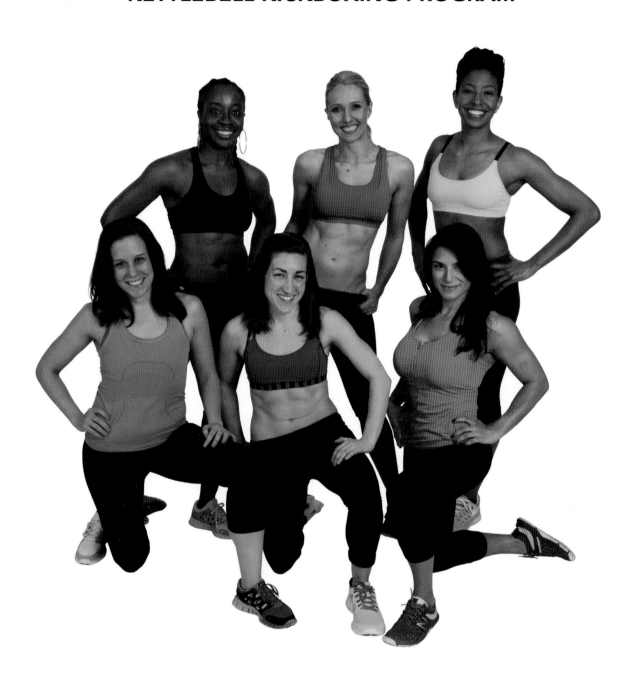

You probably picked up this book for one of three reasons:

One: you've been seeing kettlebells (not "kettle-balls") in your gym, on television, at your friend's house, and even in home goods stores. Honestly, you'd just like to know what the hype is all about.

Two: you feel a bit "stuck" in your current fitness routine, and you've heard that kettlebells are great for both cardio and strength training, they do wonders for abs and glutes, and they burn triple the calories of other weights. Now you want to know how much of this is really true and how you can get in on the action.

Three: you grabbed this book because you already train with kettlebells, and you are sold on them, but you realize that you are only scratching the surface with all the kettlebell possibilities and workout options. You love the bell; now you just want more!

In the end, no matter the reason, one thing stands true: as women, we all want the same thing out of our workout routines. We want the opportunity to find the very best of ourselves and our bodies. We want to train smart and have fun training, and we want to leave the training floor more energized, clear-headed, and happy than when we got on it. When you dedicate yourself to a healthy lifestyle, you want all the benefits that come with it: a lean, strong, feminine body that is both functional and capable. Luckily, the combination of kettlebells and martial arts is the perfect tool that can be used to accomplish all of these goals. For busy moms and professionals, it is nice to know that a kettlebell workout can function as both strength and cardio, providing a perfectly balanced routine in under an hour. For those of us interested in a fitness challenge, the kettlebell works balance, agility, mobility, flexibility, power, strength, coordination, speed, and breathing; there is always something to strive toward.

Welcome to this wonderful journey of discovering your body and making it fit and healthy for life! Although you might be working toward a specific health or weight goal, I hope this journey far surpasses those first few goals and becomes an integral part of your life pursuit of health and wellness. You may find some of the concepts, facts, and programs here simple, while others may seem challenging. I ask that you rid yourself of any doubt here and now and keep an open mind. You have already taken the most difficult step: picking up a program. This program will help you restructure your understanding of wellness, build a real foundation of health, and achieve incredible, measurable results.

MY STORY

It can be hard to take the advice of a fitness professional—after all, when it's someone's day job to stay in shape, their path to fitness isn't exactly relatable. But I'm here to tell you that I wasn't always fit and healthy, and I have experienced firsthand the difficulty of balancing school or a nine-to-five job with a health and fitness program. Though my journey to get to this point was not easy, it has resulted in a wealth of knowledge from trial and error, as well as a great deal of research once I found the right path—all of the benefits of which you can reap with this program.

About ten years ago, I lost about forty pounds . . . but that is just a small part of my fitness struggles!

When I turned fourteen years old, almost twenty years ago, I began to gain weight. It came on fast and continued all through high school and then college. It was a tough transition, to say the least, going from being comfortable with myself to feeling like a lazy outcast.

I think the worst thing about a change in weight is having to define yourself all over again, when you look in the mirror at the reflection of a person you no longer recognize. Suddenly I hated jeans, shorts, dresses, and the dreaded bathing suit. When I look back now, I am not sure how I gained so much weight so suddenly: a breakup, puberty, a lack of sports programs in my school, stress over college, stress over getting my first job afterward . . . the point is that I hated the way I looked in the mirror and how I felt every day. I had a lack of energy, a lack of confidence, and a lack of control. I was unhappy with myself.

Making Changes

By my last years of college, I knew I had to take action; if not, my entire life would be spent feeling like I didn't belong in my own skin. To start, I visited a few gyms, but I had no clue how to work out. I could not afford a trainer, so eventually I settled on my first systemized workout: a strength and cardio workout DVD I could do at home. Soon I began to see and feel a difference.

Seeing It

I remember clearly the first day I saw my abdominal muscles in the mirror. More importantly, I was full of energy and life; I was active and strong, and through that I had found a whole new meaning to my goals (many that were outside the gym).

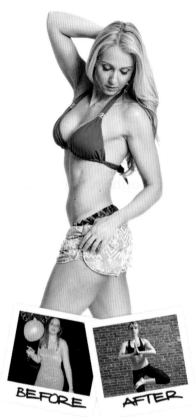

*Results may vary from person to person

Turning Progress into Pain

When I had finished college and moved to the city, the change of pace and the new responsibilities set me off of my routine. I began following a random schedule of gym visits and workouts with no structure. Shortly after that I began to gain weight again. I was stressed. The fear of gaining weight back loomed over me constantly. I began to compensate by skipping meals and undereating, sometimes not eating at all and other times overeating from stress. Suddenly my strong and defined shape became weak. I no longer had muscle definition or a healthy glow . . . instead, I was constantly exhausted and stressed about food and exercise. My healthiest habits became my biggest points of stress.

By my early twenties, I knew I needed an intervention. In many ways I had come so far, losing weight, becoming active, and building the body I wanted. After college, I had lost my regimen, and the fear of gaining weight threw me into a spiral of poor habits: yo-yo diets, lack of structure in my training, and unsustainable nutrition habits. Committing to an actual program of training was the only way I had achieved true results. That was my first lesson in fitness, and returning to it would make it clear: I had to start over.

In my initial research I realized that there was an abundance of self-serving information out there. When I tried to learn about fitness, I constantly felt like I was being sold on a gimmick. When I tried to learn about simple good nutrition, I was being sold a fat burner supplement. When I tried to figure out a way to train my body, the things I found left me spending hours at the gym—an hour for cardio, an hour for weights, and a different hour for functional training, flexibility, and high-intensity workouts. It was too much.

It took time to regain the trust I once had in myself—to find the patience to train, eat, and live correctly. I think the toughest thing was finding the balance between hard work and smart work. I had to learn to trust my routine again, trust my eating, and trust myself. It took years of dissecting information, reading research studies, and, of course, testing what worked.

Full Circle

It was that journey that helped me make the decision to leave a corporate job and go back to get my master's degree in sports science. I was and still am determined to help others find **a better way—a *lifestyle*, not a diet. A *program*, not a workout. A *habit*, not a trend.** I realized that keeping a lean and strong healthy body is sometimes more difficult than building one. People get obsessed with keeping their results and become tangled in a web of useless or bad information. They try to go above and beyond and become exhausted, poorly fed, and overtrained. In developing Kettlebell Kickboxing (KB), I wanted to put together all of the tools that truly worked for me. I had to learn to trust that what I was doing was enough—and that trust came from the perfect combination of kettlebell exercises and martial arts motion. The workout engages all of the major energy pathways needed to burn fat and still build lean muscle. It uses both traditional and brand-new exercises.

It took another decade of testing KB before this book was born. I saw the results and the effectiveness of the maintenance of KB on my own body, and after offering my DVDs and classes and seeing the results on countless women from all over the world, I was convinced that the program can work for everyone. It's fun and has enough variety to keep it that way—even when performed several times a week. Kettlebell Kickboxing is designed to help you achieve and maintain your incredible results.

MEET YOUR TRAINER

Today, I have a master's of sports science and specialty trainer certifications with two sports science associations, plus a variety of extra certifications in various areas of my field. I am a martial artist, and I have written fitness articles for magazines and trained celebrities. I am considered a fitness expert. I not only develop programs for movie actors and performers, but I also work with real women daily in my sold-out NYC classes. I have been written about in *Self, Shape, Fitness, Women's Health, Cosmopolitan,* and *Vanity Fair.* Credited as an expert at transforming the female body, I developed this program out of my passion for fitness and martial arts. I truly believe that women can and should have the opportunity to feel strong and sexy. I have produced and developed three fitness DVD series, including the nonweighted (no kettlebell needed) *7-Day Lean Series* and nutrition program, the *Scorcher Series* (kettlebell or dumbbell) four-disc training set and clean-eating guide, the two-disc *Scorcher 2.0 Series,* and the eleven-disc kettlebell *Body Series* DVD set and nutrition guide. I am also proud to be a part of NASM, ACE, and AFAA, as well as an NSCA continuing education provider, where I offer KBI and KBIA (kettlebell instructor and Kettlebell Kickboxing instructor) certification courses accredited under each of these organizations.

YOUR PROGRAM: KETTLEBELL KICKBOXING

So what is Kettlebell Kickboxing?

Kettlebell and Martial Arts—a Perfect Combo

Kettlebell Kickboxing is the one-of-a-kind fitness method I created and developed that combines the efficiency, diversity, and versatility of kettlebell workouts with the fluid movements of martial arts, including Muay Thai, kickboxing, Brazilian jiujitsu, and karate.

> For more on why the kettlebell is the most efficient workout tool, you'll find a full discussion of kettlebell benefits in chapter 1.

Some KB routines include intervals of moves that are solely martial arts moves to break up a kettlebell workout. Other moves combine kettlebell and martial arts and are only found in the Kettlebell Kickboxing program (one of many in this book is the jiujitsu sit-up). The KB program uses martial arts motions for mobility, cardiorespiratory, strength, agility, balance, and flexibility training; however, we are not learning martial arts outright—we are just using many of the benefits of martial motion and combining them with traditional kettlebell science and strength training to make a very unique and complete workout.

The mantra of our program is simple: **science, efficiency, and fun**. Kettlebell Kickboxing was designed with physiology, biomechanics, and sports science in mind. It provides a solid strength and conditioning routine that builds fundamental movement patterns, enhancing the functionality of each set of moves and workout as you progress. The martial arts portion helps us add a heart-pumping yet low–joint impact routine that encourages a deep level of mobility and balance, while the kettlebell allows our program to include strength and power as well as a low-impact yet highly challenging cardiorespiratory workout.

Why combine kettlebells with martial arts?

Because of the variety of motions, movement patterns, and energy pathways that can be engaged with the kettlebell, modern martial artists were some of the first to truly appreciate the kettlebell and place it in their strength and conditioning routines.

Martial artists are always looking for high efficiency. They are also looking for tools to complement and enhance their training and goals. Martial arts movement is fluid and natural, with a wide range of motion.

In my research, I found that tracing some of the movement patterns of martial arts with kettlebells led to the greatest results in all of our test subjects, as well as in my own body. We have seen masters deep into their seventies still practicing the motions of martial arts, and the same is often true of kettlebell practitioners as they age. Since longevity is often overlooked in trendy, high-intensity routines, I find it important to circle your training back to what matters most—building, strengthening, and preserving the body, *not* breaking it down.

HOW TO USE THIS BOOK

No matter who you are, what your fitness level is, or how familiar you are with kettlebells, I want you to remember the lesson from my story—a fitness plan doesn't work unless you stick to one complete program. There are many ways to use this book, but keep that message in mind and make a commitment to your program.

If you're new to kettlebells or haven't worked out in a while, this will be a challenge, but I welcome you and applaud you for making this change in your life. It's a big step, so be sure to inform yourself so you're comfortable before you try any of the moves or programs for yourself. Think of this like a cookbook—before you start cooking, you need to read the whole recipe so you know if you have all the ingredients and can make a plan so you don't have to keep checking the recipe and risk burning the meal. Before you start a move or routine, be sure to understand all of the guidelines so you don't risk injury.

If you've worked out with kettlebells or kickboxing before but are new to this program, you have some of the tools—but even if you're a weight-lifting trainer or martial arts master, this is a whole different ballgame. Refamiliarize yourself with the sports science behind what you're about to do, even if you might have done it before—with so much contradictory training advice and styles out there, there's a lot here specific to this program that you might be surprised to find out! Be sure to check out our special guidelines to the swing, which is often taught incorrectly. And don't miss out on the rules for your training in chapter 3—they will keep you going and help you stick to the program to get unbeatable results! This is a program unlike any other, so even if you know some of the sports science behind it, it's important that you start this program with the intention to follow it.

If you are already a Kettlebell Kickboxing fan, you may already know some of the information in this book from our class, DVDs, or blog—treat this as the bible to your program. Read it through to check that you're on track mentally and physically—you might be surprised to find your form or attitude could use some refreshing to take your KB workout to the next level! The step-by-step chapters 5 through 8 will break down some of what you've seen but never had the chance to spend time studying outside of class or the fast-paced DVDs. This book is yours, so go ahead and write in it—fill in your goals and body measurements to check up on your progress, mark up what plans you want to try in chapters 10 through 12 ("Burn 500," "15-Minute Workouts That Work," and "Your 4-Week Plan"), and get the most out of your Kettlebell Kickboxing workout! You know it works—and now, it's as if you have me as your personal trainer whenever you want to flip this book open!

This book teaches the correct body mechanics for some of the most fundamental yet misunderstood exercises. Once you've mastered the basics of the program from chapters 1 through 4, you can choose to skip over to chapter 5, 6, 7, or 8 to target an area of the body that troubles you most (such as your abs or legs)—read over the exercises and then pick one of the three unique workout plans at the end of chapters 5–8 to do at home or at the gym. You can also choose from the total-body workouts from chapters 10, 11, and 12.

EXERCISE, ATTITUDE, AND YOUR GOALS

Before we can start, I would like to have you answer two crucial questions.

The following two questions are essential to my health and wellness approach, and I believe that without understanding and addressing both, you cannot attain or maintain a healthy and balanced body and mind.

The first question is personal: **What limits you?**

The second question must be answered and understood before you move forward with training: **What is exercise**?

So, let's go on and discuss both.

Question One: What Limits You?

Having worked in the health, fitness, and martial arts fields for over a decade, I can honestly say that one of the biggest hurdles holding people back from lasting success is a limiting belief system. We achieve what we believe we can. That our bodies are not just bound by the reflection we see in the mirror. That we have the capacity to move and build new motion and strength.

So, before we continue any further, I would love for you to join me in a little exercise.

Let's begin at the end. How do you see yourself at the end of the next seven days? At the end of the next four weeks? How about six months from now? Take a moment and visualize it.

Here's what I think you see: a stronger, more mobile, slimmer, and healthier you. You have tighter muscles, a flatter stomach, a glow of energy, and a feeling of empowerment. You're less stressed, more in control, and perhaps even more focused. You're more confident in your fitness routine and nutrition choices. You trust yourself and your body.

You're right about all of it. You will look, feel, and live more confidently. Exercise and healthy sustainable living cause infectious positivity and self-assurance, traits that will seep into other parts of your life!

Now, picture your program:

Three key factors compose your complete program. We will discuss each separately and then link them together to create a lifestyle. The three components are habits, nutrition, and fitness.

Your habits are the components of your day and your personal values. I don't mean work or family; I'm referring to the individual qualities pertaining to *your* mind, body, and spirit—no one else's.

Your nutrition is not to be confused with a "diet." Nor is it to be confused with an occasional indulgence, like birthday cake or Thanksgiving dinner. Your nutrition includes what you put into your body as well as the healthy daily routines that allow you to enjoy your food and feel satisfied.

Your fitness is your basic daily regimen: working out on a program with specific, measurable, and attainable goals. Your workout should help you build bodily strength, mobility, flexibility, and balance with the added benefits of weight loss, lean body composition, and good health. Fitness should also help you become pain-free and energized.

Through this program, you will learn how to seamlessly combine all three factors to create a real lifestyle for yourself—one you can enjoy forever, have fun with, and easily maintain.

So, now that we've visualized it, let's get started and make sure that you are limitless.

Question Two: What Is Exercise?

Now that we have identified your goals and mentally worked past any and all limits, it is important that we work through the next question: *What is exercise?* Now, I understand that this may seem elementary, but many people answer this question wrong. In order to get the body you want, this must be the very first thing you understand.

This might shock you, but exercise is not sport. Marathon running, swimming, playing tennis, basketball, and even surfing and martial arts like kickboxing are sports, but they are not a strength training and conditioning exercise routine.

There is sport and there is exercise—the two are very different. The reason we often confuse them is that in the modern day, many people have taken up recreational sport activity as a way to stay active and fit (most times using this sport as a form of "exercise"). However, sports are not your exercise routine—recreational sports are your "activities," "sports," and "hobbies." Your exercise routine is the strength and conditioning regimen used to get you in shape for your sport and to help you fortify your body and avoid injury from your sport, as well as in your life. *So why all the confusion?* Let's face it—the word *activity* is bland, while a word like *exercise* merits respect amongst our friends and peers. When I say I exercise, it means that I have discipline, I am strong and healthy, and I care about myself. Activity, on the other hand, could be a random act of anything. You might still be confused—I know I once was. I thought that people who go and play basketball with their friends or run marathons or box are exercising—but no, they are being active, and perhaps they are recreational athletes, or even professional athletes. But if you notice, even marathon runners, swimmers, football players, and all other athletes have a strength and conditioning exercise routine exclusive of their sport.

There are two reasons to follow an exercise program:

Performance enhancement: a solid exercise program is meant to improve your ability in a specific sport. This is why triathletes, basketball players, tennis players, swimmers, and all other professional athletes take part in a regular, regimented, and prescribed strength and conditioning routine.

Injury prevention: as you train, work out, or exercise (all interchangeable terms), you are fortifying and balancing your body. Correct exercise should never lead to injury. While minor injuries can be common when playing a sport, it is absolutely *not* okay to get hurt lifting a weight or a kettlebell or doing a push-up; the latter (the exercises) are made to fortify your body and aid injury prevention.

> **FIT FACT:** Exercise should never cause injury. Properly conducted, exercise will instead make the joints and connective tissue more mobile, as well as increase your ability to exert more force. Proper exercise will improve performance and longevity in any activity or sport you do, and do the same in your life.

The byproduct of exercise is a healthy and fit-looking body. Yes, I said the byproduct! While many of us take on exercise to lose weight and look better, in the true definition of the term, improved body composition and increased cardiorespiratory functioning is a simple byproduct of fitness and exercise. And while you can also lose weight and feel better when you become active and perhaps begin to take part in sports, exercise is directly related to balancing the body and providing the best overall results in health and wellness.

So why is the information in this introduction so vital for you to understand? Personally, if we are training together, I believe that we should be transparent. You should not simply follow my every move or every word, but be educated on why you are doing the exercise and what benefits you will gain from proper training. Another reason is that I will need your trust. Just as I asked you to trust yourself, I will ask you to trust the program.

I also believe that the people who get and keep the most results are those who have a clear understanding of what fitness is. In this book I will be laying out a plan for you. Many of the exercises will be unique and fun, and they will challenge you both physically and mentally. But I want you to understand that as diverse and unique as I try to make your experience, the basics of the workouts will always rely on the fundamentals of fitness.

And Lastly, No Excuses!

Fitness is for EVERYONE: younger and older; pregnant (with a doctor's consent); men and women; people who are inactive, deconditioned, and athletic; celebrities, you, your neighbors, and your friends alike.

Find time to work out. You can use this book anywhere: at the gym, at the beach, in a park, in your hotel room, or at home. Many people prefer to train at home. It saves time, and if the routine is done correctly it can be as effective as the gym. Your workout must be free from stress. It should aim to build your relationship with yourself. Your workout time should be your sacred time. This is why we provide thirty- and fifteen-minute workouts in this book; *no excuses* means fitting it in and taking time out for yourself. Don't worry, fifteen- to thirty-minute workouts can be just as effective and efficient as your longer training sessions.

A Historical and Modern Look at the Culture of Sitting

In the 1900s, people worldwide were active between six and ten hours a day. Today, most of us make our livings with our minds instead of our bodies. We drive to work, we drive to run errands, and we often drive to our weekend outings. We sit all day at work, and we also commonly entertain ourselves by sitting. It seems natural, but it's not. Our bodies are designed to move. In truth, the more we stay static, the more we are hurting ourselves, becoming sedentary, weak, out-of-shape, uncoordinated, and fat individuals.

Our bodies are made and designed to move. To push, pull, crawl, walk, jump, squat, hinge, throw, turn, twist, stretch, kick, run, hop, roll . . . we are made for this—but when was the last time you did any of those things? (Be honest!)

A survey by the Institute for Medicine and Public Health revealed that adults spend an average of approximately **fifty-five hours a week sitting in a chair,** whether they're watching television, using a computer or tablet, driving, or reading.

Worse still, women are often more sedentary than men because they tend to hold less physically active jobs than men do. It's also common for women to spend less of their leisure time playing sports, especially when they get older. Having said that, to succeed, you need an approach that's built around the modern lifestyle; you also need a result-proven approach, one that works with time constraints and your individual needs. The moral of the story here is simple . . . for all of the reasons just listed and for all of your own personal goals, you have no right *not* to train your body. You have no right not to move your body and explore all of its amazing potential. Your body, if you let it, is truly limitless. Set it free!

YOUR BODY

Let's identify your current measurements. Then you can continue to evaluate your progress not only on the scale, but also in the way you look and feel. Keep in mind that when it comes to tracking your progress, the first and most important factor is your health, and then how you function and feel; your strength, energy levels, and mobility matter most. After that is the way you look in your clothing (and out of your clothing, of course!), and only after that should your weight matter.

Identify Your Goals

Identifying your goals is the first step. To begin, review the body fat diagrams that follow and answer the following questions: Where are you now? Where (safely and realistically) do you want to be in four weeks? In eight weeks? Six months from now? How about this time next year—would you like to have maintained your results?

Invisible Goals

It is important to note that not all of your goals will be, nor should they be, aesthetic. In the chart that follows, some common areas of imbalance and dysfunction are identified. It is important to figure out your points of weakness and pain, as well as your imbalances. Then you can create a game plan with a solid and balanced strength and conditioning routine to cure such issues.

Body Fat Percentage

Using the body fat percentage diagrams, do the following:

1. Look at yourself in the mirror.

2. Honestly identify your body fat estimation based on the silhouettes in the diagrams.

3. Remember, this is you today—if you want to change something, you can and you will. The human body and mind have amazing potential.

For women:

- 10–12% body fat is essential.
- 13–20% body fat is considered a healthy range for athletes.
- 21–24% body fat is healthy for fitness.
- 25–31% body fat is still considered an acceptable range.
- 32% body fat or more is considered obese.

It's completely okay to embrace your desire to look better no matter what percentile range you fall into! It is perfectly okay to want to be fit in time for a class reunion, wedding, big party, vacation, or swimsuit season! After you begin working out toward your goals, you'll find that you start to enjoy fitness. You will find new challenges and goals, and believe it or not, you will miss your KB workouts if you skip them! You know why? It's because fitness, as well as your workouts, should be fun! Fitness should make you look and feel better.

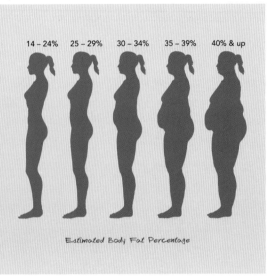

14 – 24% 25 – 29% 30 – 34% 35 – 39% 40% & up

Estimated Body Fat Percentage

MEASUREMENT TRACKER

BEFORE:

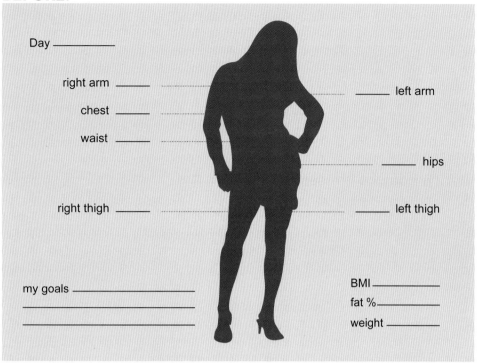

Day _____

right arm _____   _____ left arm

chest _____   _____

waist _____

_____ hips

right thigh _____   _____ left thigh

my goals _____   BMI_____
_____   fat %_____
_____   weight _____

AFTER:

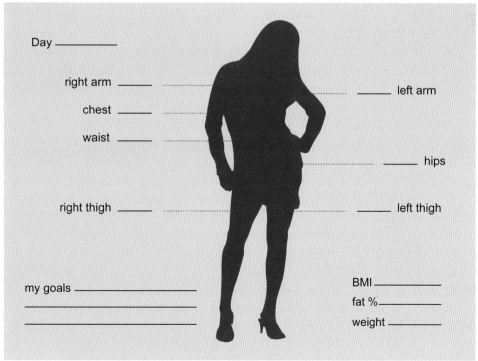

Day _____

right arm _____   _____ left arm

chest _____

waist _____

_____ hips

right thigh _____   _____ left thigh

my goals _____   BMI_____
_____   fat %_____
_____   weight _____

FACT: Fitness doesn't come from:

- Starvation
- Exhaustion
- Repetitive exercise
- Hunger
- Stress about fitness
- Suffering
- Constant sacrifice
- Pain

KETTLEBELL KICKBOXING INSTRUCTOR CERTIFICATIONS, CLASSES, AND PROGRAMS

You can always find out more about becoming a Kettlebell Kickboxing (KBIA) certified instructor on our website at www.kettlebellkickboxing.com. You can also find many of our home workout programs and DVDs there.

CHAPTER 1

THE GENIUS OF THE KETTLEBELL
The Sports Science Behind the Kettlebell

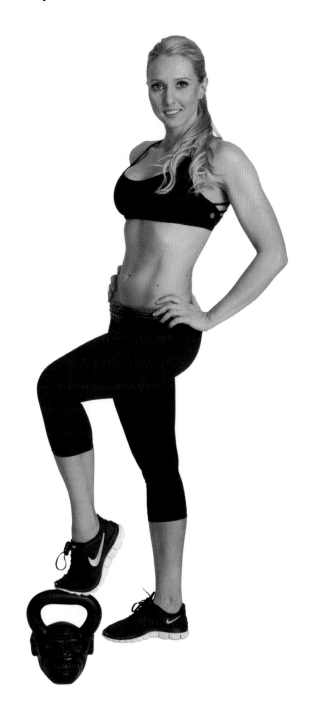

1

A decade ago, the popular concept of women's fitness included a great variety of classes, books, advice, and workout DVDs; kettlebells, however, were not on that list. Today, that has changed dramatically. Kettlebells have been featured in many ad campaigns by successful companies selling women's fitness clothing, and the most popular gyms carry kettlebells. Celebrities like Jessica Biel, Jennifer Lopez, Pink, Penelope Cruz, Kim Cattrall, Megan Hilty, Jennifer Aniston, and Kim Basinger are speaking out about their love for kettlebell training. It can even be argued that more women are picking up the trend than are men.

Why? It's simple . . . women are smart. We know how to recognize a good thing when we see it. We love efficiency. We have no time to waste. Women want more! We want to cut our training time in half, challenge ourselves, and see real results both aesthetically and physiologically. In our quest for more efficient ways to get in shape, women began to hear tales of shorter, more effective, result-driven, functional, low-impact workouts with something called the kettlebell.

THE KETTLEBELL?

According to a 2010 American Council of Exercise study, twenty minutes of kettlebell exercise burned an average of 272 calories. That's expending a phenomenal 20.2 calories per minute, the equivalent of running a mile in six minutes.

It's simple; kettlebell exercises burn more calories in less time compared to more traditional workout regimens. One of the reasons is that training with a kettlebell requires you to engage multiple muscle groups. Kettlebells also can be used in unique motions that are classified as **ballistic**, meaning they are of a higher intensity than other weight-lifting motions (known as grinds, which will be explained in chapter 2) and can produce the same effect on the body as sprinting, running, or jumping (but with far less impact on the body and joints—when executed correctly).

> **HERE'S A BONUS:** If you're stuck in a crowded gym with lines to the machines, a kettlebell has no waiting time! Just pick it up and go. With kettlebell swings, you can achieve a similar cardiorespiratory effect and calorie burn as a three-mile run, with the added benefit of strength training.

Kettlebells have been around for centuries and have roots in ancient Europe. There is much debate as to when and where kettlebells originated, but the first recorded mention of the kettlebell, known in Russian as *girya*, was in a Russian dictionary in 1704. Some historians say that the concept of the kettlebell dates back to Spartan times, when men would put wires in cinder blocks and swing them for exercise.

Interestingly, long before kettlebells became a popular exercise tool seen in most gyms, cast-iron balls were used as standard weights for trading throughout Europe. Although kettlebells disappeared from this everyday use, they resurfaced in the realm of entertainment, used by strongmen, or *gireviks*, to demonstrate their abilities by lifting and throwing the iron spheres in circuses, markets, and fairs.

As time went on, so did the evolution of the kettlebell. In czarist Russia, kettlebells were completed with a handle and began to emerge as a primary tool for Russian strongmen. In the twentieth century, the Soviet army used them as part of their physical training and conditioning programs.

In the United States, the kettlebell has had a rebirth—it's in TV commercials, pop culture, gyms, and group classes. Two of the most notable trainers responsible for the popularization of kettlebells are Pavel Tsatsouline and Steve Maxwell. Today kettlebell training is for everyone! Just look at the wide assortment of kettlebell colors and weights found at online retail websites and in fitness stores across the country—from black to blue, orange to pink, kettlebells today are available in weights ranging from 5 to 105 pounds.

> *Did you know?* **In fitness, anything you can do with a dumbbell you can do with a kettlebell; however, everything you can do with a kettlebell you cannot do with a dumbbell. See chapter 2 for more on substituting a dumbbell for the kettlebell.**

IF YOU ARE GOING TO TRAIN WITH THE KETTLEBELL, YOU NEED TO UNDERSTAND IT. SO, HERE'S YOUR KETTLEBELL CRASH COURSE!

> Read on . . . we'll teach you how to get rid of knee pain and train your legs sexy without bulking up the quads—yes, all that with the unique versatility of the kettlebell!

Engaging the Forgotten Muscles

The kettlebell is able to train and engage the **posterior chain** like no other kind of workout. The posterior chain is a group of muscles including the glutes (buttocks) and hamstrings that are commonly inhibited when sitting. As we stand and begin to do exercise, the muscles do not fire (work/engage) correctly during actions like squatting, lunging, running, or simply walking up the stairs. Only when you execute the kettlebell swing correctly—using only the posterior chain (as we will show you in chapter 4)—do the forgotten and inactive muscles have to fire and reactivate! This is truly vital to the balance of your body and its kinetic chain. It is also very important for anyone looking to improve sports performance, including faster and more efficient runs. This helps avoid knee overuse due to muscle imbalances, and for all those women sick of bulky thighs and the lack of a shapely behind, posterior chain motion like the kettlebell swing will engage the muscles in the backside, teaching them to work during other motions like the squat or lunge, and helping to get more shape and less quad (front of the leg) bulk. *Why else do you think we love the kettlebell so much?*

Safer Training

Kettlebell workouts use ballistic motions (such as swings) to produce the same cardiorespiratory effect on the body as more impact-driven (and often injury-causing) exercises like high-impact plyometrics such as box jumps, knee tucks, and other sports science techniques that should be reserved for professional athletes with individualized prescriptions and supervised settings. This is crucial to understand, because sports science has found that not everybody should be jumping on boxes and doing high vertical jumps (just to name a few high-liability plyometric motions), especially not if they have muscle imbalances. Doing these motions too soon on a deconditioned or untrained body will leave you overtrained and injured—if not directly after a workout, then most definitely over time. When swung using the correct form, time interval, and weight, the kettlebell can more safely produce the same cardiorespiratory and physiological response as the potentially dangerous plyometric moves many people do at the gym.

The Postworkout Effect!

Exercise was traditionally placed into two categories: strength training and cardio. There is so much more that can and should be discussed regarding both of these terms.

The term *cardio* is often interchangeable with *aerobic exercise*, generally a steady-state, low-to-intermediate-intensity exercise regimen that uses fat as its energy fuel—which is a quicker-burning fuel than carbs. Examples include jogging, fast walking, hiking, using an elliptical machine, or taking a slower-paced aerobics class. While this form of exercise begins to use mostly fat as fuel approximately twenty-five minutes into the workout, it has little effect on fat burning after the exercise is done.

In contrast with cardio, *strength training*, or *anaerobic exercise*, has an incredible metabolic effect on the body after the session is complete and for a potential twenty-four to forty-eight hours afterward. Another benefit of strength training is the lean muscle your body builds; this muscle starts to eat away at the fat, because muscle tissue is more metabolically active and therefore requires more energy (calories) to live. Basically, when you have lean muscle tissue, your body burns more energy, or calories, throughout the day—it's a wonderful byproduct of strength training and your Kettlebell Kickboxing exercises.

REMEMBER: Just doing cardio alone will not give you the lean, strong, and versatile muscle tissue you want. To get fit and look lean, you need strength training!

The beauty of Kettlebell Kickboxing is that we will tap into both forms of training in one workout. Our martial arts intervals will keep your body active and moving throughout the entire workout, while the kettlebell and body weight strength motions will help build lean and strong muscle tissue. Another benefit of KB? Once you have learned the program in this book, the kettlebell will help you build more lean muscle and get all of the benefits of the postworkout effect, where the body will be metabolically more active, helping burn more calories and build lean muscle mass that will be taking the place of fat.

For all of these reasons, kettlebells have an edge over other workouts! *So, are you ready to meet your kettlebell?*

CHAPTER 2

KETTLEBELL 101
Anatomy of the Bell

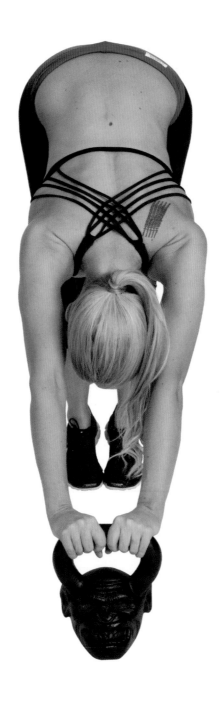

To train with the bell, you should understand its anatomy—and yours!
Unlike more conventional training equipment such as dumbbells or weight bars, the kettlebell's center of mass is extended due to its unique shape. The kettlebell's ball and handle structure helps create the ideal grip and weight distribution for ballistics.

Because of the shape of the kettlebell and its unstable force, the core is engaged throughout every motion. This, in conjunction with the posterior chain activation and safe yet challenging ballistics, makes the kettlebell a truly valuable yet often misunderstood and underused tool. This book will open your eyes to all of the possibilities of kettlebell motions as it teaches you to execute them and maximize every one of the many benefits. We have a great variety of kettlebell movements here, and while of course there are more than what's in this book, the ones provided here have the most versatility and usefulness.

MEET YOUR KETTLEBELL

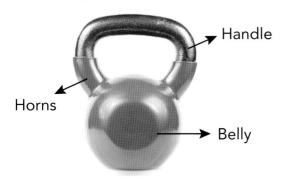

Handle

Horns

Belly

In settings that use kettlebells very traditionally, you might actually see/hear the term *pood* mentioned. A pood is a Russian unit of measuring weight. It is sometimes even listed on the kettlebell itself. This means that the kettlebell is a standard 35 lb weight.

HOLDING POSITIONS AND GRIPS

Racked Position

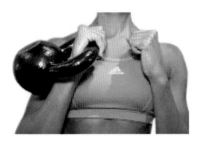

Hold the kettlebell between your shoulder and forearm on the outside of your wrist. Your elbow should be bent and tucked right above your hip, while your wrist is straight and strong (no bending of the wrist) and your thumb is touching right in front of your breastbone. Traditionally, you would clean the kettlebell to this position.

Double–Racked

Hold two kettlebells in the same way as described above.

Mid-Racked

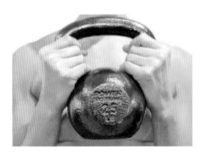

Hold the kettlebell between your shoulder and forearm inside your wrists with both hands, gripping from the horns (the very bottom of the kettlebell handle). Always keep the kettlebell close to the body, elbows in, with a strong, straight back and at chest level. Your elbows should be bent and tucked right above your hips, while your wrists are straight and strong (no bending of the wrists).

Goblet

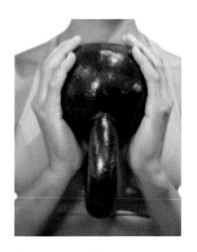

Hold the kettlebell between your shoulders and forearms at chest level—by the belly of the bell, not by the handle. Your elbows should be bent and tucked right above your hips, while your wrists are straight and strong (no bending of the wrists) and your thumbs are touching right in front of your breastbone.

Bottoms-Up

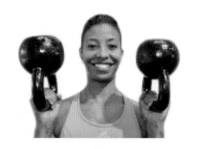

Hold the kettlebell upside down by the handle. This can be done with one arm or two, at a racked position or overhead, depending on what the move calls for.

Bottoms-Up by the Horns

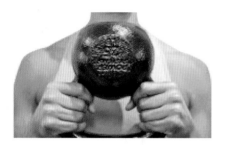

Hold the kettlebell in a mid-racked position, but upside down, so that the belly of the kettlebell is above, not below, while the handle faces down. Still hold at the horn of the kettlebell, and all mid-racked rules apply.

Hanging

With the arm extended down and in front or to the side of you, depending on the move, your shoulder should be packed into the back and not hanging. The back should always be straight with good spinal posture. Engage your glutes and core. This can be done with one arm or two, depending on the move.

KETTLEBELL TERMS

You may have picked up this book for the workouts alone, but I stand by the fact that the more you know and understand exercise, especially the tools you will be working with, the more you will be able to answer your own questions and the less likely you will be to fall for misleading or bad information.

Kettlebell motions are distinguished in two forms: **kettlebell grinds** and **kettlebell ballistics**.

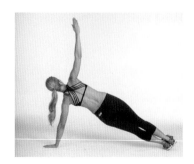

Kettlebell grinds—any exercise used to develop strength. Grinds are exercises you can also perform with a dumbbell and are usually done slowly with fewer repetitions. An example of a grind is a squat, press, bicep curl, or lunge.

Kettlebell ballistics—exercises done where the kettlebell is in motion and you are using your posterior chain and momentum to generate the movement. Ballistic movements are usually used to develop power and speed and are done at a high number of repetitions. These movements increase power and endurance while incorporating anaerobic principles. An example would be the kettlebell swing. Most kettlebell ballistics are done from a hip hinge, not a squat.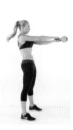

Most people, and even trainers, get this part wrong! Kettlebell ballistics are the most difficult motions to understand—most people squat or lift the bell instead of generating the power from the hips. KNOW YOUR FORM! This is key.

Your Anatomy and Its Part in Kettlebells

To understand the kettlebell and its unique ability to shape, reshape, and help build and balance the body, we must look at our own anatomy.

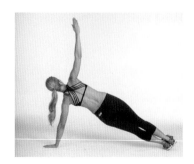

The **posterior chain** is a group of muscles, tendons, and ligaments on the posterior kinetic chain of the body. I sometimes call these the "forgotten muscles" because it's easy to forget about what you can't see in the mirror, and these muscles are often neglected in other workouts. Plus, due to our sedentary lives, the more we sit, the more this area of the body becomes dormant and forgets how to work during movement.

Most importantly for kettlebells, the posterior chain includes the muscles of the hamstrings, glutes, and back. The muscles that make up the calves and other muscles that run along the back of your body are also included in the posterior chain. In ALL of your kettlebell swings, you will be using this set of muscles.

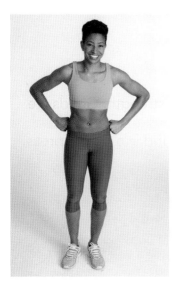

The **anterior chain** is made up of the muscles that sit in the front of the body: the chest, shoulders, quadriceps, abdominals, and biceps. I like to call these the "beach muscles" because they're the ones we worry about people seeing when we lay out at the beach.

Most of us go into the gym, look in the mirror, and work the muscles we see; our arms, our abs, our obliques, and our legs. Many women might also work the glutes, but often by doing quad-dominant motions like lunges and squats. What most of us miss is the correct way to train the posterior chain. Kettlebells accomplish this through the swings and all of the swing variations that we'll show you in later chapters.

Kettlebell Motions

The last few terms you should be familiar with when picking up the kettlebell are the positions from which you will be using the bell, either as moves or as transitions between moves:

Rectilinear—motion in a straight line. For kettlebells, this means lifting in a straight line perpendicular to the floor.

Curvilinear—motion along a curved path. This means swinging the kettlebell in a variety of ways.

Styles of Kettlebells

Many people don't realize that there are two styles associated with kettlebells.

Hard Style: more traditional kettlebell movements in which you use a large amount of body tension throughout the work phase of the exercise, expending a great deal of energy with each movement. The focus is on building strength, improving body awareness, and correcting imbalances by breaking down an exercise movement to its simplest form to generate efficient movement patterns. It sets the foundation for soft-style training.

Soft Style: also called *girevoy*/fluid style, used in the competitive sport of kettlebell lifting where you try to expend as little energy as possible throughout the work phase of the movement so you can manipulate the weight over long periods of time and a large number of repetitions.

KETTLEBELL WEIGHT

Okay! Now that you know your way around a kettlebell, which kettlebell should you choose? Yes, these guys come in all sorts of colors and even designs—including the monkey kettlebell my husband got me for Valentine's Day. But, all kidding and fun aside, kettlebell weight is extremely important. In many motions it will also differ significantly from the weight you are used to with dumbbells, so please listen up!

Correct Weight for Kettlebell Ballistics

Because most kettlebell exercises, excluding simple movements such as a bicep curl or presses, are compound, or multijoint, motions, you need to pick a kettlebell that is the correct size. **Remember that not all exercises are created equal**—if you take a five-pound weight and use it to do a kettlebell swing, you will NOT get the benefit of the swing.

In kettlebell ballistic motions like the swing and all of its variations, if you pick a kettlebell that is too light, your first instinct will be to lift the kettlebell with your arms, and since this is the direct opposite of what a kettlebell swing should be, you won't receive any benefit and can even hurt yourself with incorrect biomechanics. And even if a weight that is too light is correctly distributed across the posterior chain and core, the weight will not be enough to get a desired response from the body.

Other form issues with using light bells for ballistic exercises include squatting, backward bending, and not engaging the glutes or the entire posterior chain.

When picking a kettlebell, especially for your swing, it MUST be a heavier weight than you can lift forward in front of you comfortably with your arms.

As a woman, you should start your swing no lighter than a twenty-pound kettlebell and progress to a weight of thirty to forty pounds. Kettlebells between twenty-five and thirty-five pounds are the choice for many Kettlebell Kickboxers in our classes.

Correct Weight for Kettlebell Grinds

For grinds, which include traditional forms of exercise such as presses, curls, squats, and rows, you might want to consider having one or two weight options that are typically less than your kettlebell ballistics weight.

Our General Recommendations:
- New to exercise/deconditioned: 10, 12, or 15 lb kettlebells for grinds PLUS your 20–25 lb kettlebell for swings and ballistics
- Intermediate/active: 15 or 20 lb kettlebells for grinds PLUS your 30–35 lb kettlebell for swings and ballistics
- Advanced/highly trained/kettlebell-experienced: 20 or 25 lb kettlebells for grinds PLUS your 35–45 lb kettlebell for ballistics

Please note that it is entirely possible and okay to swing a kettlebell over 45 lbs. Many women who are familiar with the standard kettlebell double-handed swing use 50, 55, 60, and even 70 lb kettlebells.

To help you make an educated choice, see the following chart of desired effects and reps.

Standard Sports Science Information

A **set** is the number of times you will be doing an exercise or a specific combination of exercises.

A **rep** is the number of repetitions you will be doing in a specific set.

Rep range dictates how your muscles adapt and react to your training, and in turn what type of results you can receive from your workouts.

Ways to Train: Reps or Timed Intervals
1–3 max rep—Power Training
5–8 max rep—Strength Training
8–10 max rep—Hypertrophy (building muscle)
10 and up—Muscle Endurance and Fat Burning
Time Intervals, HIIT—Fat Burning
(Time Intervals can be a mix, but typically they work Strength Training and Muscle Endurance)

Double kettlebells! If you double the kettlebell, you can double the fun— and the intensity—of the training.

- **All of the exercises that require double kettlebells will be shown and noted.**
- Make sure that your kettlebells are of the same size and weight.
- What you can do with two kettlebells, you can always still do with one, so don't worry if you don't have two kettlebells.
- You are adding more weight to the mix by doubling up on kettlebells, so pay extra attention to form.
- Generally, double kettlebells are just a bit more advanced than doing the move with a single kettlebell, but if you follow the step-by-steps in this book, you are good to go!
- When picking a double kettlebell weight, consider starting with two 10 or 12 pound kettlebells and then working your way up to two 15 or 20 pound kettlebells.

- Please note that many of the exercises here will be done for time intervals.
- When I say max rep, I mean that you should pick a weight you can lift up to 8–10, or 5–8, or 1–3 reps, meaning you pick a weight heavy enough that you would not be able to go over that amount. Therefore in an 8–10 set you would pick a weight heavy enough that you cannot go over that tenth rep.

Keep in mind that the numbers in the chart are standard, but you should play around with getting to know your body every few weeks. Try to change up the reps slightly; play around between eight to fifteen reps to see what might work best for your body.

In this book, the workouts will be prescribed to you, and you can simply follow the plan!

CAN YOU USE A DUMBBELL?

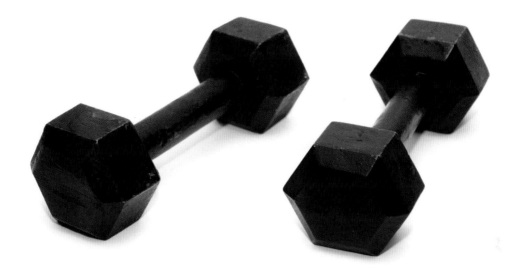

Using dumbbells with this program is actually okay! Yes, the kettlebell has a better structure, and ideally you should be using a kettlebell with the program. However, I'll give you some guidelines that will help you to substitute a dumbbell if a kettlebell is not available for your workout.

For grinds, it's easy to sub in a dumbbell if you don't have a kettlebell handy because the weight is fixed in your arm and does not have to be swung. Get used to holding the dumbbell where it is most comfortable and becomes a part of your body. Make sure to position the dumbbell in exactly the same area of the body where the kettlebell is positioned in each picture.

Ballistics, or swinging motions, require more care if you're going to use a dumbbell instead. The kettlebell has a handle and is made to swing easily, but a dumbbell has no handles, so you must pay great attention to your grip.

When you swing the dumbbell, hold it by either the dumbbell handle or by the top of the weight, depending on what is more comfortable. Make sure you are using the exact same motion and biomechanics as described with the kettlebell.

The kettlebell clean might be the only motion that is challenging, because the dumbbell cannot fully rest on your forearm; perform the clean exactly as described, but instead of resting the dumbbell on the forearm, grip it and hold it tightly packed to the body, the same way you would in a racked position.

TRAIN SAFELY

Of course it is vital to note that you can't simply do as you please in fitness—because your spine can only bend and twist so far, you should only do the exercises and movement patterns your body can do. You must follow the rules of biomechanics and avoid any movement with or without the kettlebell that challenges the natural patterns and abilities of the body. While it is completely true that our minds and bodies can push past many barriers, in your fitness routine, those barriers should never compromise the health of your body.

RECAP AND REMEMBER!
1. Never compromise form to finish a set or a workout.
2. No one knows your body better than you do. If something feels wrong, it might be, so stop and rest, or just stop the motion.
3. Pushing hard is great—but pushing too hard, too fast, is not. Take your time and study each motion. If you go slow, you'll still get an amazing workout and become a pro in no time!
4. Pick a smart weight.
5. Form first!
6. Train both posterior and anterior chains.

CHAPTER 3

BALANCE YOUR BODY AND MASTER YOUR MIND

Breathing, Finding Your Fat-Burning State, and Fighting Your Limitations

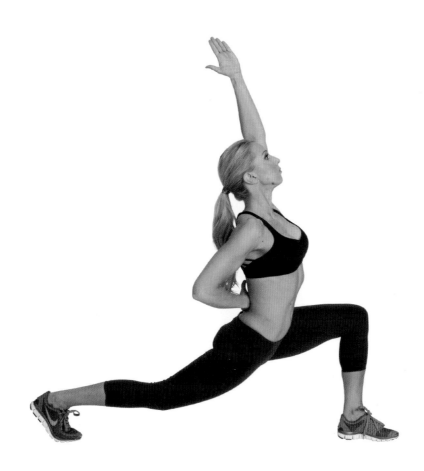

Before we begin our training, it is important that you understand a few of the concepts covered in this chapter. Specifically, I want to further discuss two key factors in the mental portion of your training: habits and limitations. I will also discuss and explain a few physical factors, including correct exercise structure, breathing, and fat burning, as well as general rules for efficient training.

TO SUCCEED, YOUR MIND AND BODY MUST BE ALIGNED

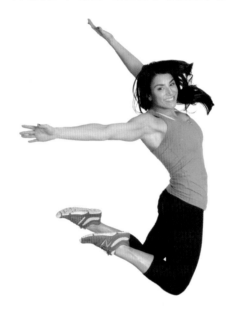

Forming habits is the key to your success! You can have the best intentions and the greatest goals and dreams, but if you don't establish good habits, then none of these things will matter. I have a basic saying, and I believe in it: Good habits can make us great. Poor habits can break us down.

The good news? Studies show that human nature *loves* habit. If you give yourself the chance, your body will embrace your new routine. If you give yourself the chance, your mind will be less stressed about "getting things done," "getting your workout in," and "eating healthy." Why? Because these practices will become habitual. You won't think about them, and you'll have more time for real things, like family, friends, work, and hobbies. Plus, much of what you learned through the Kettlebell Kickboxing program will also apply to other aspects of your life! Here's how . . .*

---

*   For those who already own my DVDs and training programs, these five factors of habit may look a tad bit familiar; however, I believe that in every program the five factors listed must be repeated, because these are the very factors that can make or break your success.

1. **Identify your bad habits.** *(We all have them.)* Figure out what it is you want to change. Identify it, write it down, and hold yourself accountable. Realize that this is you today, but tomorrow you can do and change anything you want!

2. **Decide to change these things.** Identifying and making a decision are two separate things. It only takes twenty-five days to establish a good habit, and that's no time at all considering the full course of your life, health, and happiness. Go for it! Let's decide to change some things.

3. **Create a path to change.** Read on to help you figure out the processes you need to create to help you achieve your full potential.

4. **Follow through for twenty-five days, and it becomes your new habit!** Just remember the habits you will have formed once you have followed this program for twenty-five days. You will have made and seen changes in your body you never thought possible! Today is day one.

5. **Let's create a path to change.** Trick yourself. If you want to watch less television and read more, studies have shown that the best way to accomplish this is by hiding the remote control and placing a book on your coffee table instead. The idea is simple: make things easy and accessible. How? For example, if you want to learn to speak Japanese, you may choose to erase all of the music on your phone playlist and download Japanese 101 to listen to during your daily commute instead. You just made learning Japanese much simpler. Think point A to point B.

   Creating a path to change is often about tricking yourself by making good choices more available. Basically, place the things you want right in front of your face while hiding the alternatives. For example, if you drink ten coffees a day, get rid of all the coffee in your home and don't carry spare change when you leave your house. Go as far as taking a different route to avoid your favorite pastry or coffee shops. Allow yourself one ritual coffee in the morning, and then stock your work fridge with coffee alternatives, like natural green tea. Announce your new habit to others so that friends can hold you to it. Finally, reward yourself after you establish your good habit. For example, for every full week that you have successfully followed your training charts, take yourself out to your favorite sushi restaurant on Friday as your treat. **Remember: Creating good habits is evolution. Maintaining poor habits is deterioration!**

BALANCING YOUR BODY

Once you learn the sports science behind exercise and health and fitness, no one can ever sell you on false science, false products, or an injury-prone program.

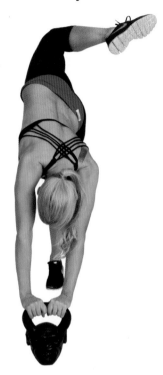

I would like to truly explore the definition of exercise from the introduction of this book. I understand in the beginning you might have picked up this book to have an encyclopedia of new kettlebell and martial arts moves to add to your gym routine, home workout, or fitness class. However, I hope that this book gives and teaches you so much more. So, let's start by balancing both your body and your fitness knowledge.

When you train, you have goals—and no matter whether they include weight loss, strength, speed, a leaner body, mobility, flexibility, or sports performance, your program must fit your body type and your desired effects. The program must also address your specific weaknesses. Those weaknesses could be from a lack of strength, development, or mobility, as well as from old injuries and bad habits. A training program is only as good as it is able to cater to your physical goals in a progression that also helps fix, not mask, any weaknesses. Additionally, it should be both attainable and maintainable.

Many people start down a bad path at the very beginning. People tend to lay fancy fitness routines on top of their weaknesses. In other words, some have poor movement patterns and weak, tight muscles, yet instead of working on a basic and balanced routine to fix this, they begin to perform high-level motions or high-impact sports on top of these dysfunctions. That, my friends, is like placing brick on top of sand; in the long run, it won't hold up.

No, all hope is not lost! This book, as you will see, has unique motions and awesome combinations of exercise and time intervals, all of which will make your training fun, challenging, and progressive. However, we will always go back to the basic movement patterns—the core of correct workout structure and progression.

All of our training will include the following foundational skills:
- Pushing—vertical and horizontal

- Pulling—vertical and horizontal
- Squatting—this includes countless variations
- Hinging—hip motion, including but not limited to the kettlebell swing
- Locomotion, rotation, and transverse motion

If there is a push, there must also be a pull. If not, then your body will become imbalanced, overdeveloping and overworking in one area while weakening in another. If you do a push-up or a press, you should also do a pull or a row.

Most people have huge difficulty with the hinge—and the hinge is the primary motion of the kettlebell swing! The hinge is difficult for many people because most of us sit for so much of the day. By sitting, we inhibit muscles, and they become inactive. Not being able to hinge properly means not being able to properly engage the posterior chain of the body, particularly the glutes. Instead, many kettlebell users try to use their knees and lower backs to do all the work. It's no wonder that knee replacement surgery has overtaken hip replacement surgery as the number one procedure of the baby boomer population.

Squatting is more complex than it looks. While almost anyone who exercises knows how to squat, many people do it too often and incorrectly, working only the quadriceps in lunges and squats. Without activating their glutes to avoid weakness, these people are left with knee pain when performing a basic movement pattern like the squat. By waking up and strengthening the glutes and entire posterior chain in hinging, you'll find that squats become pain-free and beneficial in myriad ways.

Locomotion: let's think of this as movement. You can move and get all of the benefits of working with your body with very safe drills and exercises. Instead of performing crazy jumps and reckless plyometrics, we will include locomotion like kicks, calisthenics from different martial arts, pivots, SAQ (speed, agility, and quickness) drills, and other safe and highly beneficial ways to put the body in motion.

RULES FOR YOUR TRAINING

Here are a few of my basic training rules. If you choose to ignore these, you will get only a fraction of the results this program offers. We might take some of these things for granted—a clear mind, mental focus, or a program—but when you want to see results, these little factors can be the defining keys to your overall success.

- When you train, it's key that you detach from the rest of your life and focus on reconnecting with your body and mind. Your workout can and should become your own daily oasis. Revel in your tired muscles and sweat! No one can take your hard work and determination away from you.

- Do not skip modifications to some exercises if you aren't yet familiar with the move, have never worked out before, or haven't trained in a long time. A few exercises, such as the push-up, show a modified version. You'll still get all of the benefits with the modified versions!

- If you feel overwhelmed at any point, please stop whatever you are doing and take a moment to breathe before jumping back in!

- If you miss a day, a few days, or even a week, do not stress over it. Just keep going! If you only missed a day, start with the following day's workout. If you've missed a week, pick up where you left off.

- If you feel pain, go back and reevaluate your form. If you feel like you've overtrained, take a break. Soreness doesn't win you any medals!

- Be patient! Good program design (exercise and nutrition program combined) always yields results. Each person's body reacts differently, and some people will see results faster than others.

- While your physique is important, don't just fixate on how you look. Be proud of your body's strength and mobility too!

- Intensity is what matters! However, intensity only makes sense when your form is correct. Never get to a point where you are actually breaking your body down.

- Lastly, remember how great it feels to work out and accomplish your goals. This is how you deserve to feel every day. Your family, friends, and coworkers also deserve to have this version of you in their life. Plus, you'll inspire them!

BEFORE YOU TRAIN, YOU MUST ASK YOURSELF:
- How is this helping me?
- Am I following a program?
- How does this affect my joints?
- What am I training for?

Once you have answered these questions and been honest with yourself, you can continue with the knowledge that the time you are taking out of your day to exercise is directly improving your body, your mind, your spirit, and your health.

FAT BURNING

There is a lot of information out there about burning fat. Unfortunately, with that information also comes a lot of misinformation. Often people highlight only a portion of science in order to sell you something. The basic fact is that if it seems too easy—like "eat this and get that in one week"—then it is probably a con, often something that is dangerous for your body or simply not true.

In my own fitness journey, I have often wished for a quick fix, but in reality the only way to get rid yourself of fat and keep it off is to include strength training and clean eating in your life. That is it! With that said, you don't have to be on a diet, and it's okay if you don't swear off cake. Nor do you have to lift weight every single day for two hours a day. By following the program in this book, you will burn fat; that, my friends, is a given.

BREATHING

When you breathe correctly in your training, your lungs become stronger, you have a better "filter" in your body, and you are able to absorb more oxygen and gain more energy.

Why does breathing play such an important part in your exercise? When you breathe incorrectly during exercise, get stressed, or don't sleep enough, your adrenal glands release the stress hormone cortisol. That response, which is meant to give you a burst of energy for fighting or fleeing, causes you to accumulate and store fat in your belly. Sustained stress can keep cortisol production at high levels and leave you craving high-sugar and high-carb foods.

Poor breathing during exercise can put your body into a state of panic and cause your body to hold onto fat as you exercise. Don't panic! Simply follow these guidelines:

- Breathe in through your nose and deep into your belly. Breathe out through your nose or mouth.

- *Never* gasp or gulp for air with your mouth. If you find yourself doing this, decrease your exercise intensity and maintain a slightly slower pace that matches your breathing.

- If you're struggling with your breathing, try this old martial arts drill: take a sip of water and do not swallow it during your entire high-intensity set. Good! You just taught yourself not to breathe with your mouth.

The more in touch you are with your breath, the more you will achieve from your workout. If your goals are clear, and if they connect to your body through your breath, you will see results manifest quickly.

> If you can't breathe correctly, you won't burn fat to your best potential.

KB Strategies for Success

Strategy #1: Rethink Your Standards

Adjust your standards and adjust your role models. Don't look to your friends and coworkers and people just like you when determining your standards. Look to people who are highly successful at what they do. Do not talk to your best friend about what she did at the gym; look at the girl doing push-ups instead (unless, of course, your best friend is the one doing those push-ups!). Read stories about athletes. Read biographies of incredible human beings. Aspire to be like your favorite athlete. Look to someone who is successful to be a role model. Set your standards higher than your local peer group. Think you can't "do that"? Be un-reasonable. Be crazy. Aim beyond your own expectations! Why not? What do you have to lose—and what could you gain?

Strategy #2: Fake It—Till You Become It!

The second strategy is to fake it. When trying to help yourself overcome self-imposed limitations, trickery may be the best tool. Tell yourself, "I have time" (even if you don't). "I have energy," even if you feel tired. "I have will," even if you feel like you don't. "I have strength and ability and power and I will suc-ceed." FAKE IT till you BECOME IT! That's what all the greatest people do; I do it every single day—join the club!

Strategy #3: You Become Who You Hang Around

Surround yourself with people who are better than you—that's a rule. Surround yourself with people who work harder and who have more dedication than you do. Surround yourself with people who inspire you. Read about, follow, and engage with people who inspire you. At the same time, cut the people, shows, hobbies, and routines that hold you back—trust me, it will feel amazing after you do it. If you are always surrounded by those you are better than, there will be no motivation to improve, no reference point. You will become stagnant. You'll set lower goals for yourself and you'll find yourself limited. Find people who challenge you, motivate you, and help push you to become better. Condition yourself to be better!

Strategy #4: Set and Always Reset Standards

Have you ever heard a person say, "I just beat my personal best" or "I just crushed my record"? That is a personal goal—and it is important that you set goals for yourself in every aspect of your life, fitness included. Do not just set a goal weight. Set goals for the number of push-ups you can do in one minute, the number of swings, the weight of the kettlebell. Set goals for the number of sprawls or squats, or the length of your plank. Track your progress in weight and take notice when a heavy weight become easy to lift. Set goals on how technical you are about your form in your movements. By setting and reaching and readjusting your personal goals, you will break free of self-imposed limitations. BUT— do not rush! Your first goal should always be great form and proper technique.

IT'S GO TIME

Okay, now I believe that you have all of the tools for success. All you have to do is turn to the next chapter and begin to learn and follow the Kettlebell Kickboxing program.

See you on the training floor!

CHAPTER 4

SWING YOUR WAY TO A BETTER BODY
This One Motion Can Transform You

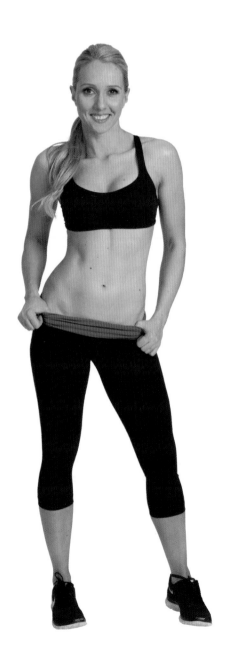

No pressure—but the swing is a rite of passage in the kettlebell world. We'll start with the double-handed kettlebell swing. To get all of the unique biomechanical benefits of kettlebell, this motion must be executed correctly. This is the foundational exercise to all of the ballistic motions you will be performing with a kettlebell.

WHY SWING?

Do you remember in chapter 3 when I discussed the movement patterns we should all incorporate into our routines: push, pull, squat, hinge, and locomotion? Well, the swing is beloved for its hinge. I find that most people have tremendous difficulty with the hinge, and this is because they spend most of the day sitting. The inability to hinge is linked by our culture of sitting to the reason many of us suffer back pain, knee pain, and weakness. Not being able to hinge means not being able to properly engage the posterior chain of the body, particularly the glutes. Without hinging, the same muscles that help you run and protect you from back weakness during many activities are now inactive. Instead, modern people and even some athletes are unintentionally using their knees and lower backs to do all the work their butt muscles are supposed to do. This leads to overuse and misuse of other areas of the body, and this leads to knee pain and eventual knee and ankle injury, as well as back pain, which can then lead to shoulder and neck injury.

> In sports science we call using a muscle "firing" a muscle, while the terms "muscle imbalances" and "inactive or weak muscles" mean not being able to fire a muscle during a motion where that muscle is required.

The kettlebell swing is all glutes, all of the time! When you swing the kettlebell correctly in any swing variation, you engage the posterior chain, fire the glutes and hamstrings, and strengthen the areas that have been weakened or deactivated by day-to-day sitting. If you have any of the pain or imbalances associated with not being able to hinge, the kettlebell swing is a perfect weapon to use to wage a war on them.

Yes! The kettlebell swing can help eliminate back and knee pain!

More reasons to love the swing!

As we learned in our kettlebell anatomy, the swing is a ballistic motion. Not only does this posterior chain hinging motion help us complete a hinge in our training and balance out our body, but it also teaches us to fire muscles and help us correct muscle imbalances in our favorite sports and activities. The kettlebell swing is also an incredible and super safe metabolic conditioning tool. It can help burn triple the amount of calories burned in a more one-dimensional training regimen!

You might not get it right away, and that's okay. I find that it can take students one to three class sessions or DVDs after initially being taught the swing to get it, so be patient with yourself. Remember that these are muscles and movement patterns that have not been worked in a while. Once they begin to work, you are now firing your glutes and hamstrings and reactivating them, or teaching them to work and pitch in during simple motions like walking, running, jumping, kicking, lunging, and squatting.

So, let's swing!

As discussed, the swing is the basis of all kettlebell ballistic movements. It starts with **a hinge, not a squat**—this is very important. In a hinge, the bend in your hips comes before the bend in your knees. Hinging also means you should bend your knees to a lesser degree than that of your hips. Do not squat! You will be swinging the kettlebell from behind your knees, with your grip above your knees. Remember to bend more at your hips with a slight bend at your knees and a straight and strong back. You will be incorporating your posterior chain and momentum to generate the power of the movement. As a result, the kettlebell should feel almost weightless when it comes up to the terminal position of shoulder height. Squeezing your glutes at the top of the motion, you should be standing straight and upright with hips forward and knees straight (there should be *no* overarching of the back) at the end of the motion.

The kettlebell should swing between and behind your legs and up to shoulder height in a nonstop, repetitive motion.

TRADITIONAL DOUBLE-HANDED KETTLEBELL SWING, STEP-BY-STEP

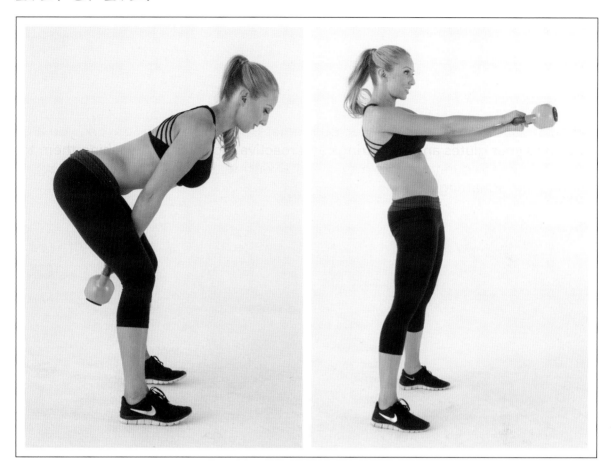

1. With both hands, pick up the kettlebell by the handle and sit back in a hinge, bending first and more deeply at the hips, then at the knees.

2. From the hinged position, swing the kettlebell back and behind your knees.

3. Swing the kettlebell up to shoulder level with your arms straight as you thrust your hips forward and raise your torso back into the standing position.

   - Make sure your butt muscles are engaged by squeezing your glutes together tightly.

   - Do not raise the kettlebell with your arms. Your arms and the kettlebell should feel weightless through the entire motion.

4. At the top of the swing, remember to keep your arms straight, thrust your hips forward, straighten your knees, and swing the kettlebell no higher than chest level as you rise to a standing position.

   - Do not bend back at the top of the motion.

SWING YOUR WAY TO A BETTER BODY

5. Continue without stopping back down into your hinge and repeat steps 1–4. Create a nonstop fluid motion of the swing, with the kettlebell going behind the knees and back up to shoulder level.

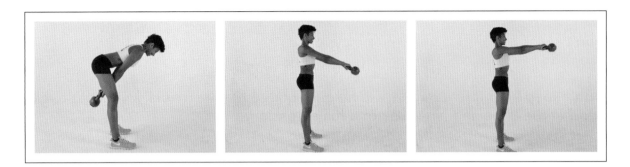

Notice how everyone's swing is slightly different, but the hinge remains a constant!

FORM

- The first thing to understand with kettlebells is that you must link your body together into one strong chain of action. This principle ensures that you will not be placing too much pressure on any one joint or muscle. Additionally, it will secure the total-body principles on which kettlebells are built. Link your body by applying proper form, checking your alignment and center of gravity, and executing each move with a flow of motion.

- Stay rooted into the ground. Never explode out with the kettlebell and find your heels or toes off balance or off the ground. In swinging motions especially, keep yourself rooted and remember to engage the glutes.

- In your swing, **do not squat!** Generate power with your hips by pushing your hips back toward the wall behind you (not by squatting to the floor) and then snapping your hips forward.

- Do not hyperextend or bend your back into a backward bend. Your glutes must squeeze together before you can even attempt a backward bend.

- Aim to squeeze your glutes before the kettlebell reaches face level—as it does, pop the hip forward and consciously let the kettlebell fall back behind the knees.

- At the hinge, the kettlebell falls above and behind the knees. At the standing position, it comes up to face level and no higher.

- Speed comes from making sure your force and body drop the kettlebell down, not letting gravity do all the work.

Don't squat! If you squat during this motion, it will not be a posterior chain motion, therefore you won't be focusing on the glutes and hamstrings—the very area this motion was created for! Remember—a squat is a squat and a hinge is a hinge!

Don't lift the kettlebell with your arms! You can easily hurt yourself, *plus* this is not a lift or an arm exercise. The kettlebell should feel weightless in your arms the entire time.

Don't keep your legs straight. The hinge required for a kettlebell swing has a mild bend at the knee and hip—it's not a full extension.

Don't backward bend. Remember that your butt muscles are supposed to stop the motion of the bell at the top. If you let the kettlebell go past your shoulders and you do not engage the glutes, you risk hurting your back instead of strengthening your back, core, and butt muscles. So make sure to stop at shoulder level, and keep your glutes activated and protecting the back. Your butt muscles should not allow a backward bend.

REMEMBER: All of your swinging motions will come from this form, so practice this and try to execute each step as instructed. If you are not following the protocol, you are not doing a kettlebell swing, and you are not getting the benefit. So no squatting or arm lifts; use your hinge and the power generated by your hips as well as the stability of your core—nothing else!

> *MOST common mistakes: You are NOT squatting. You are NOT raising the kettlebell with your arms. At no point is the swing an arm- or quad-dominant motion. It is all hips and core.*

The kettlebell swing requires a hinge, not a squat.

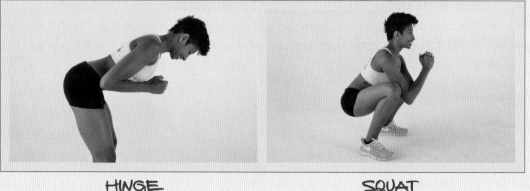

HINGE   SQUAT

PLEASE NOTE: Throughout this book there will be many variations of this swing, but the roots will always be the same.

When I say **"using your swing technique,"** I mean that you should use the exact same technique that is described and illustrated here.

How to Use the Swing

Once you learn this motion, you can easily place the swing as a set or an interval into your circuit or regular workout. You can even do the swing on its own for a perfect strength and cardio workout! A perfect combination would be swings and push-ups, paired with squats or lunges. Believe it or not, this is a very complete combination of exercises.

But considering the fact that you have this book, you don't have to worry as much about workout structure. Everything will be listed out for you. Your only job is to pay very close attention to form and to show up and do the work I lay out for you! That's it.

Now that we have learned the swing, we will incorporate it into our training as a cornerstone of many of the chapters and workouts.

If you have not tried it yet, I urge you to get up and try it! Make sure to follow every step listed.

To warm the body before these two swing workouts, aim to warm up the body for five minutes, using one of the basic warm-ups from chapter 9.

Try this solo swing workout:

TABATA SWING WORKOUT

- Set a timer for a 20-second work/10-second rest period—and set it to 8 sets (4 minutes total).
- Now, following perfect form, as described earlier, swing the kettlebell for 20 seconds, and rest for 10 seconds. Continue that for 8 sets.

MILESTONE SWING WORKOUT

- Set a timer for 1 minute, and with good form begin to swing the kettlebell.
- Count your swings.
- Remember the number as you rest for 30 seconds.
- Swing again, this time aiming to beat your last number by 2.
- Rest again for 30 seconds.
- Swing again, this time aiming to beat the last number by 2.
- Form first! Do not compromise form for an added rep. If your form is wrong, that swing rep should not count!

HIIT? That stands for high-intensity interval training. Kettlebell swings are ideal to place into high-intensity rounds. They get the heart rate up, engage the core, work multiple muscles, and are low impact and safe on the joints.

SWING VARIATIONS

Now that you have mastered the swing, you should know that out of the traditional kettlebell swing came many swing variations. Some have been taken from power lifting and sports science, while others have been innovated by kettlebell pioneers. Several are unique to Kettlebell Kickboxing.

Types of Kettlebell Swings and Swing Options

- Double-handed swing
- Single-arm swing
- Switching single-arm swing
- Sumo swing
- High pull
- Walking swings (lateral or straight/in and out versions)
- Suitcase swing/gunslinger swing
- Swing catches
- Double kettlebell variations to the above motions

- Squat swing
- Walking squat swing
- Hammer chop swing
- Side/hammer swing

While we discuss many of these moves, we do not illustrate all of them. Many are too advanced, and are not necessary to get a great workout. Some have to be illustrated by a trainer (like the squat swing or walking swings), and they have no greater benefit than the traditional swing. Additionally, the greatest benefits can be seen from just a few of the variations of the swing.

SIX BASIC KETTLEBELL MOVEMENTS

Traditionally, kettlebell training included only six basic kettlebell movements:

1. **Swing**
2. **Snatch**
3. **Squat**
4. **Clean**
5. **Press**
6. **Turkish Get-Up**

Kettlebell Kickboxing includes many more than six moves, but it is important to know and understand the history and evolution of any art or study you choose to take part in. Kettlebells, as you can see from our brief history lesson in chapter 1, have a story, and as that story evolves, so do the motions of the kettlebell. Remember that in its earliest stages, the kettlebell was a tool used to strengthen the body for combat. It was later adapted into the performance arts and then again into physical fitness. Today, the kettlebell has found a new place in the gyms and homes of regular people who are looking for efficient ways to get fitter and healthier, faster. It is today that we see the innovations of the kettlebell swing and the varieties in kettlebell motions.

The best moves are about to be covered in this book . . . so go on, flip the page or swing a kettlebell!

CHAPTER 5

FLAT ABS AND A CAST-IRON CORE
Get the Abs You Always Dreamed Of

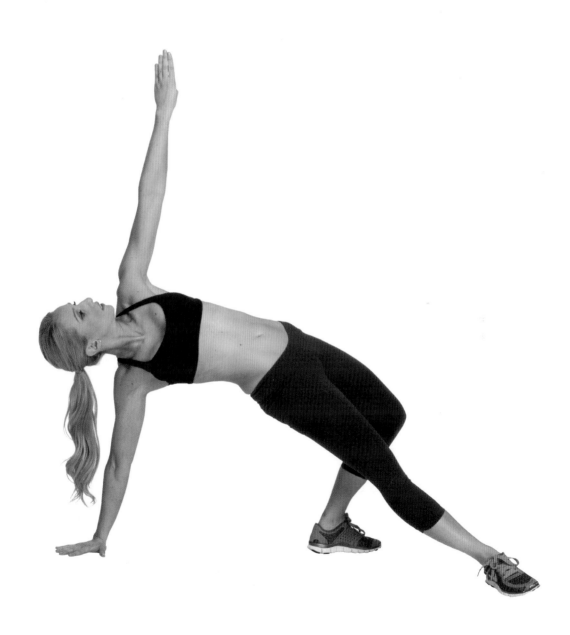

Cardio workouts alone are not enough to burn belly fat. Strength training increases muscle mass, and because muscle needs more energy to function, you will in turn burn more fat (belly fat included). This is not myth or fiction—this is fact. This is also the reason that there are so called "skinny" people with belly fat. Thus, *skinny* is not always the same as *fit*. You must incorporate strength training into your routine to get the strong core and flat abs you want. Another great way to burn belly fat is to include several high-intensity interval training sessions a week into your training regimen. Luckily, by using the kettlebell and its unique motions like the swing, as well as more standard strength motions like a kettlebell squat and martial arts moves like kicks to burpees, you'll see that your strength training and your high-intensity workouts will always include belly fat–fighting moves. Plus, the motions in this book will undoubtedly strengthen your core and improve your performance in your sport, and in your life.

> **BONUS!** Did you know that a squat can be just as efficient in burning belly fat as all those crunches? In addition to working the legs, squats are one of the top exercises for firming the abdominals and burning belly fat!

ABS AND CORE

Your core muscles go far beyond your abs. There are actually over thirty core muscles. If you work to strengthen your core, you will find a harmony between the pelvis, lower back, hips, and abdomen. You will firm the muscles in your back, obliques, pelvis, abdomen, and even butt. Your core helps stabilize the spine. It also transfers force between the lower and upper parts of the body, helping you have a powerful punch, an awesome tennis serve, or a great jump shot. If your core is weak, you can suffer from back pain and instability. Athletes with a weak core have poor athletic performance and are more susceptible to injury.

Think about it this way—your core is involved in every single movement your body does, in your workouts and in your life. Therefore, it's important for you to train it correctly and in its entirety (not just the muscles you want to see in the mirror).

Your core anatomy is composed of a few different parts, as we'll now go over.

ABS

The abdominal muscles include several important muscles that help contribute to your core's function.

Rectus abdominis: rotates and flexes the trunk of the body. This is your "six-pack" muscle.

Transverse abdominis: your deepest abdominal muscle. It helps with core stabilization and compresses the abdominal wall.

Obliques: help you bend sideways and stabilize the spine.

HIPS

Hip flexors: yes, these are actually a part of your core, and often you will feel them during your abdominal work in this ab chapter, as they allow you to flex the hip.

LOWER BACK

Erector spinae: helps with posture and stability, adjusting to maintain balance, and bending.

Quadratus lumborum: helps with posture and stability, adjusting to maintain balance, and bending.

BELLY FAT

As mentioned here, in order to fight belly fat, you must lift weights! You must also watch your diet and eat clean (as will be discussed in chapter 13).

There are a variety of reasons for why belly fat accumulates. The major culprits are lack of activity and poor diet choices—including overeating, eating poor-quality foods, and bad pairing of foods. Stress is another huge factor that many people overlook.

CORTISOL

When you breathe incorrectly during exercise, are under a lot of stress, or don't sleep enough, your adrenal glands release the stress hormone cortisol. That response, which is meant to give you a burst of energy for fighting or fleeing, causes you to accumulate and store fat, especially in your belly. Additionally, cortisol production can remain at high levels due to sustained stress and leave you craving high-sugar or high-carb foods.

- **Breathing correctly during exercise** is crucial to controlling the production of this hormone during exercise! Look over chapter 3 to make sure you are breathing correctly.

- **Stress!** Cortisol is a stress hormone, so working out, breathing correctly during your workouts, and sleeping well are all factors that can help you control this.

LEPTIN

Produced by your fat cells, the hormone leptin plays a role in appetite control. It can also slow down your metabolism! Research has found that excess body fat can cause a condition known as leptin resistance, which means your brain isn't affected by leptin even though your body contains higher levels of it.

To help avoid leptin resistance:
- Exercise regularly and safely.
- Eat clean.
- Include strength training in your workout regimen.

INSULIN

Every time you down a carb-dominant meal or drink a sugary drink, your blood sugar spikes. In response, your body releases insulin, whose job it is to pull extra glucose (sugar) from the bloodstream. Gaining weight can often lead to insulin resistance, a condition in which cells become less responsive to the hormone, as well as to diabetes.

- As will be discussed in chapter 13, eat well and pair your foods correctly.
- Avoid sugary meals in the morning, or midday sugar-packed snacks.
- Exercise or get up and move instead of drinking a soda to get a boost of energy in your day.

> Muscle burns more calories than fat! So build muscle and burn belly fat.

YOUR EXERCISES!

Your Kettlebell Kickboxing ab routine includes almost as many standing ab drills as floor work. Have you ever seen the abdominals of a martial artist? Martial artists have to have super strong core muscles in order to transfer force between the upper and lower body. Imagine how the force from your feet has to transfer to your hips and into the upper body for a punch. You don't need to be sitting or lying down to train your abdominals.

KB FIGURE EIGHT SWING

Using the fundamentals of your swing, this figure eight motion transfers the kettlebell between and behind the legs. Make sure your back doesn't round. For this move and all others, the steps may specify starting on one hand, but you can start with whichever side you prefer.

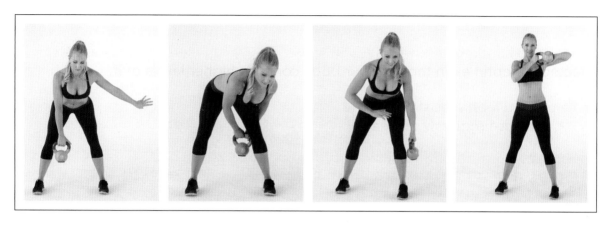

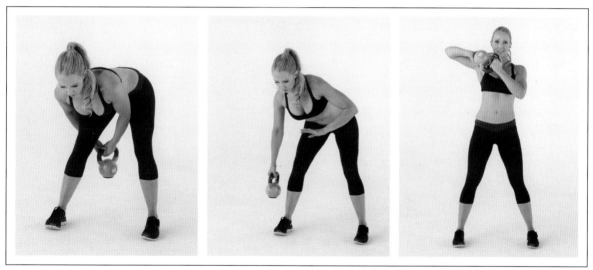

- Begin by doing two or three single-arm traditional kettlebell swings with your right hand.
- When you feel comfortable and have the swing motion perfected, swing the kettlebell up in a traditional single-arm swing. Once the downward part of the swing brings the kettlebell back behind the legs, take the left arm and bring it behind your left leg to meet the kettlebell handle.
- Grab the kettlebell handle in your left hand, switching arms as the kettlebell goes behind the legs and comes up to hang outside of the left leg.

- As you bring the kettlebell up with your left hand, bring it all the way up across the body to the left shoulder.
- Do not switch grips; just touch the belly of the kettlebell with your right hand, at shoulder level.
- To engage the back, make sure that the right hand touches the kettlebell with the inner palm, and the elbow is bent to have your right arm perpendicular to your body, parallel to the floor.
- Do not switch the kettlebell here; just touch and return the kettlebell between the legs as you would to start a traditional single-arm swing, this time with the left arm.
- At the same time, bring the right hand back behind the legs to meet the bell and switch sides, continuing the drill in a fluid, nonstop figure eight.

KB HAMMER CHOP

This is a side swing that will be moving from one side of the body to the other. Note that because this motion is categorized as a hip-dominant motion, we are still using posterior chain fundamentals, specifically the hinge.

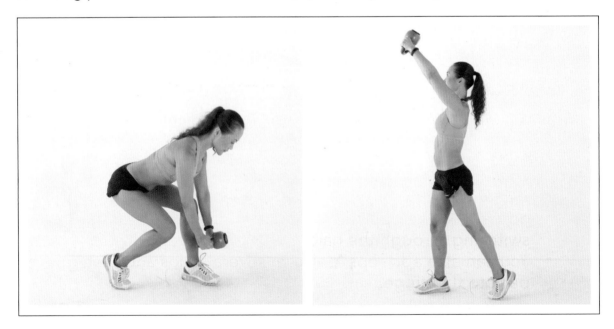

- To start, hold the kettlebell at the mid-racked position and have both of your feet together.
- As you hinge back, bring the kettlebell with you, first doing a reverse curl, and as you hinge bring the kettlebell down diagonally to your side and behind your hips.

- Remember that you are not squatting; do not twist intentionally. There will be a slight natural twist due to the kettlebell moving to one side.
- As you bring the kettlebell back up, bring it all the way up, across your body, and over the shoulder, and then back down again for the next rep.

KB HAMMER CHOP TO HALO

This is a side swing that will be moving from one side of the body to the other, like a reverse chop. Note that because this motion is categorized as a swing, we are still using swinging fundamentals, specifically the hinge.

- To start, hold the kettlebell at the mid-racked position and have both of your feet together.
- As you hinge back, bring the kettlebell with you, first doing a reverse curl. As you hinge, bring the kettlebell to your side and behind your hips.
- Remember that you are not squatting. Do not twist intentionally; there will be a slight natural twist due to the kettlebell moving to one side.
- As you bring the kettlebell back up, bring it all the way up, across your body, and over the shoulder.
- Now continue the motion and bring the kettlebell behind the body to perform a halo.
- After you perform one halo, continue back down to the chop.

The KB Hammer Chop to Halo can be performed two ways:
- The motion can be single-sided; as you perform the halo, go back to the same side each time.
- The motion can be double-sided; as you perform the halo, go back to the opposite side and continue to alternate, switching through the halo.
- You can also add reps; perform several halos and then go back to the hinge.

ADD A LUNGE for a total-body move:
- Perform the KB Hammer Chop to Halo; then, instead of going to do another set, stop the kettlebell at the mid-racked position and execute a rear lunge. (Lunge mechanics are described in chapter 7.)

SIT-UP

- Lie faceup on the floor with your knees bent and feet flat.
- Your goal, ideally, will be not to move your feet throughout the entire sit-up.
- Place your hands behind your ears, or across your chest as you hug yourself and grip your shoulders.
- You can also extend the arms out in front of you, as long as your back is strong and straight.
- Raise your torso to a sitting position, slowly and with control.
- Even more slowly, lower your torso back to the starting position.
- As mentioned, try not to move your feet or arms, and do not strain.

KETTLEBELL SIT-UP

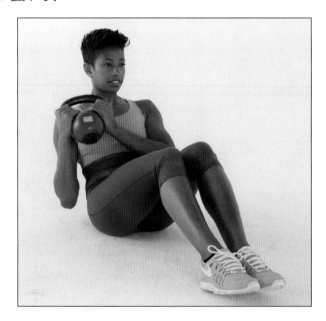

- In a kettlebell sit-up, hold the kettlebell mid-racked and perform the same motion as illustrated in the regular sit-up above.
- Keep the kettlebell close to your chest and your elbows tucked in.
- Aim not to move the kettlebell off of your chest.

> Pictured here is the side sit-up variation on the kettlebell sit-up. For the regular kettlebell sit-up, center the kettlebell on your chest.

GOBLET KETTLEBELL SIT-UP

- Place the handle of the kettlebell against your chest. Hold the kettlebell as you would a goblet (see chapter 2 for kettlebell grips if you don't remember).
- Perform a sit-up. Your goal is not to move the kettlebell handle off of your chest.

30-30-30 SIT-UP

- Complete the motion of a sit-up, but in slow-motion: take a full 30 seconds to go down, another 30 seconds to come up, and another 30 seconds to go back down.
- Keep your heels rooted into the ground and do not move your feet away from the body if you can help it.

MMA SIT-UP

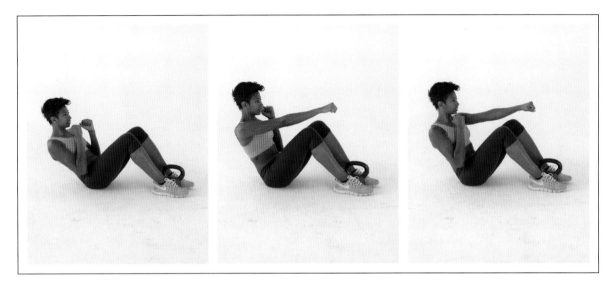

- Place a kettlebell between your feet.
- Sit down in a sit-up position.
- Clench the kettlebell with your feet as it rests on the ground.
- Begin to sit up and execute two punches* at the top of your sit-up.
- Immediately come back down and then back up again.
- Continue nonstop until your round is done.

*To execute your punches, simply hold both hands close to the chin, fists tight, and then alternate, extending the arms and turning your fists over so that the knuckle is upright. Keep your elbows in and alternate left/right (jab/cross). (For more on punching, check out chapter 6.)

BOW AND ARROW

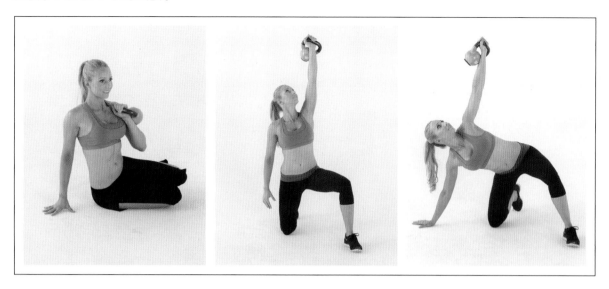

- You will start out on your knees with the kettlebell racked to one side, with your free hand on the ground behind you.

- Raise yourself up so that you are sitting up on your knees and step out the same leg as the side of the kettlebell.

- Once that leg is positioned comfortably out in front of you and you are on one knee, bring the hand without the kettlebell to touch the floor next to you as you press the kettlebell overhead at the same time.

- The arms should move simultaneously apart as if you are tightening a bow and arrow.

- Keep your eyes looking directly overhead and at the kettlebell the entire time.

- Lower back down one step at a time, just as you came up, all the way down to sitting on your knees.

- Repeat.

SIDE SIT-UP

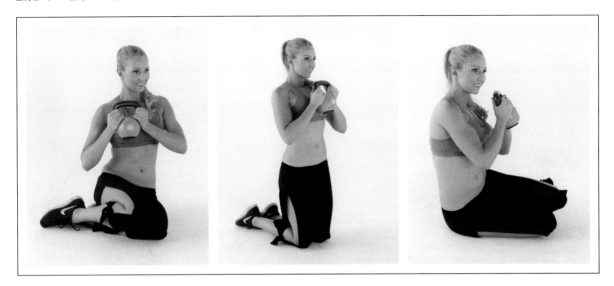

- Mid-rack a kettlebell and hold it tightly to the body.
- Sit down on your knees first, but then sit to the side of your knees.
- Holding the kettlebell to the chest, sit up all the way on your knees.
- Then sit back down. You can alternate sides or stick to one side.

If you cannot complete this motion without the help of your arm, put the kettlebell down and use your arm to help you sit up. Later, you will develop the strength to complete this motion with a kettlebell.

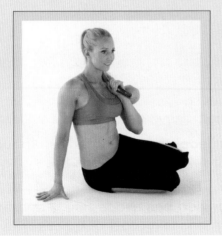

JIUJITSU SIT-UP

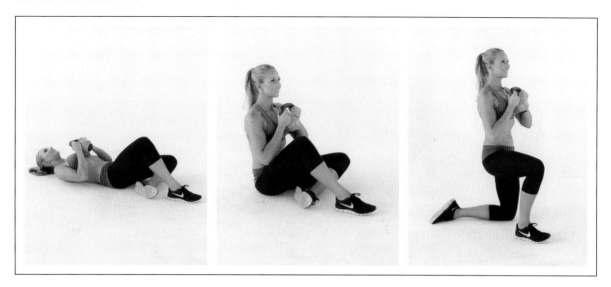

- Start off in a sit-up starting position with the kettlebell mid-racked at your chest, with one leg bent underneath the other (as in the first photo above).
- Complete a sit-up and then, at the top, bring one leg out in front of you and push onto it (see the second photo). Drive through the heel.
- Sit up, posting onto one leg and one knee (as in the third photo).
- Continue to hold the kettlebell mid-racked and close to the body as you sit back down all the way back to the starting sit-up position.

If you cannot complete this motion without the help of your arm, put the kettlebell down and use your arm to help you sit up. Later, you will develop the strength to complete this motion with a kettlebell.

JIUJITSU GET-UP

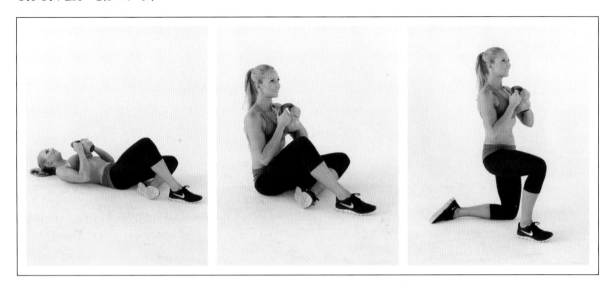

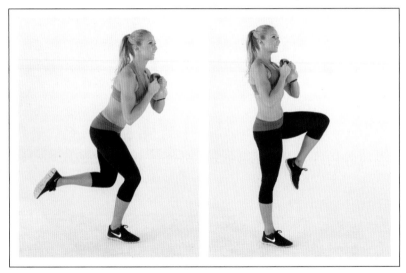

- Perform a jiujitsu sit-up. At the top, continue to drive through the front leg all the way up to a single-leg standing position.
- It should feel like you are performing a reverse lunge up.
- Drive through the heel of the foot.
- Continue back down the same way.

OVERHEAD KB SIT-UP

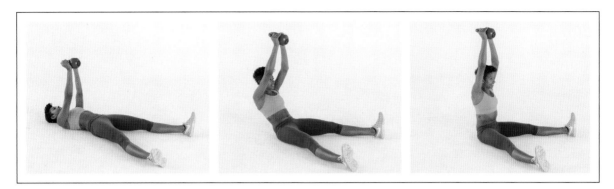

- Lay down on the floor with your feet spread apart. With both hands, hold the kettlebell by the horns and lift it overhead with your arms fully straight and perpendicular to the floor.
- Sit up, keeping your feet on the ground and your arms fixed overhead.
- As you sit up completely, continue to keep your gaze upwards. Then lower your body back down.

FORM

- Throughout the entire set of overhead KB sit-ups, your shoulders need to remain fixed, and your arms can never move.
- Your legs should be placed on the ground and your feet should be spread apart to counterbalance the weight of the bell.
- You must also be staring straight up at the kettlebell.
- Be careful not to bend the arms or extend them behind or in front of you. Until the set is done, the kettlebell must stay fixed overhead.

DOUBLE KB OVERHEAD SIT-UP

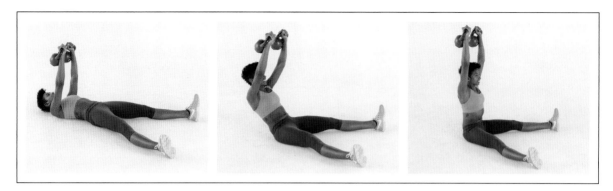

- Lying down with your feet spread apart, hold one kettlebell in each hand in the racked position (see the example of the double-racked grip mentioned in chapter 2).

- With the kettlebells racked up by the handles, extend both overhead in one steady motion, as if they were connected by a bar. The kettlebells should be extended overhead, and your arms should be fully straight. Look up at the kettlebells.

- Sit up, keeping your feet on the ground and your arms fixed overhead.

- As you sit up completely, continue to stare at the kettlebells and then lower your body back down.

FORM

- Your shoulders need to be fixed, and your arms can never move.

- Your legs should remain on the ground and your feet should be spread apart to counterbalance the weight of the bells.

- Be careful not to bend the arms or extend them behind or in front of you. Until the set is done, the kettlebells must stay fixed overhead.

KB LEG LIFTS

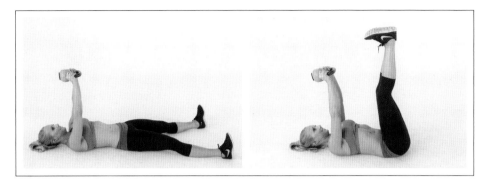

- Lie on the ground and hold your kettlebell overhead with both arms. Keep your shoulders pressed tightly into your back.
- Without moving your arms, lift your legs up so they are perpendicular to the floor. Keep your toes flexed and legs long, like you are trying to stand on the ceiling. Keep your arms fixed overhead.
- Lower your feet down to the ground, but do not rest them fully.
- Bring them back up, using your core for support and strength.
- Continue this, remembering to minimize the arch in your spine by pulling your belly button in.

KB CORE STABILIZER

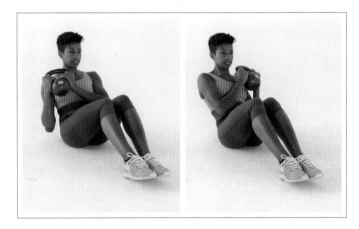

- Sit on the floor with your knees bent and hold a kettlebell mid-racked.
- Lean back so your torso is at a 45-degree angle to the floor, and make sure to keep your abdomen tight.
- Don't round your lower back, and keep your shoulders straight.

- Without moving your torso, slowly (take 2 seconds) rotate your shoulders to one side as far as you can.
- Then, slowly and with full control, turn your shoulders to the other side.
- Make sure that you turn from your shoulders, not just your arms, so that your spine is stable and all of your muscles are fully engaged.
- Pause again, then continue to alternate back and forth for the allotted time. A good goal is a set of 30 seconds.

PLANK

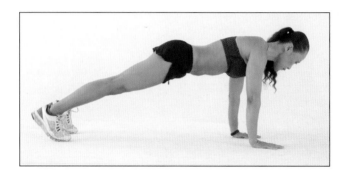

- Start out by getting into a push-up position.
- Your shoulders, elbows, and wrists must be in a straight line.
- Your body should form a straight line from your shoulders to your ankles.
- If you were to place a broomstick on your back, it should make contact with your head, upper back, and butt.
- Pull your belly button to your spine and keep your glutes and core engaged by contracting your abs as if you were about to be punched in the gut.
- Hold this position without rounding or hanging through your back. Keep all of your muscles activated.

SPHINX PLANK

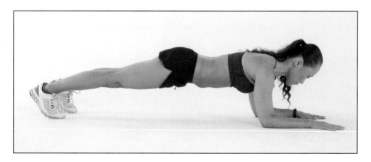

- Start out by getting into a push-up position, but bend your elbows and rest your weight on your forearms instead of on your hands.
- Your shoulders and elbows must be in a straight line.
- Your body should form a straight line from your shoulders to your ankles.
- If you were to place a broomstick on your back, it should make contact with your head, upper back, and butt.
- Pull your belly button to your spine and keep your glutes and core engaged by contracting your abs as if you were about to be punched in the gut.
- Hold this position without rounding or hanging through your back. Keep all of your muscles activated.

MODIFIED PLANK

- This modification can be performed for both regular and sphinx plank if you are having trouble with the original motion.
- Instead of performing the exercise with your legs straight, bend your knees and place them on the ground so that they help support a portion of your body weight.

EXTENDED PLANK

Once you have mastered the plank and feel like you have no difficulty holding a regular plank for 1–2 minutes, it might be time to change a variable and make the plank more difficult. The extended plank is very challenging and should only be executed once you can hold a regular plank.

This modification can be performed for both regular and sphinx plank if you find the original too easy.

- Place your weight on your hands or elbows, depending on your plank.
- Walk back with your feet, extending your plank, positioning your elbows in line with your ears. Your hands will now be farther out than your head—and farther out means the plank will be harder!

PLANK REACH-OVER

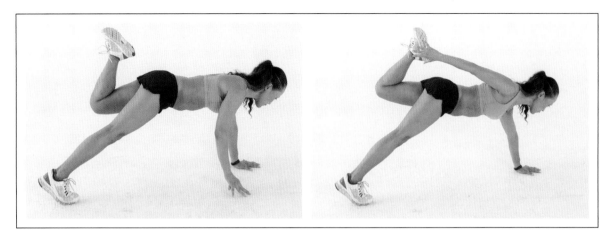

- Start out by getting into a push-up position.
- Your shoulders, elbows, and wrists must be in a straight line.
- Your body should form a straight line from your shoulders to your ankles.
- If you were to place a broomstick on your back, it should make contact with your head, upper back, and butt.
- Pull your belly button to your spine and keep your glutes and core engaged by contracting your abs as if you were about to be punched in the gut.
- After you feel stable, reach over with your right arm behind your back and at the same time kick up your left leg, touching the two while keeping maximum stability.
- Go back to the plank and hold this position without rounding or hanging through your back. Keep all of your muscles activated.
- Then continue to reach over the opposite arm and opposite foot.

How long should I hold a plank? If you have a hard time, try to begin holding for 5 to 10 seconds, rest for 5 seconds, and repeat until your time round or required set is done.

However, if you can hold a plank for longer than 2 minutes, it might be time to add a new variable. Try an extended plank, or alternate with side planks. Remember that at a certain point your body will make the necessary adaptations and you will need to change the module to keep getting the right benefit from your plank.

SIDE PLANK

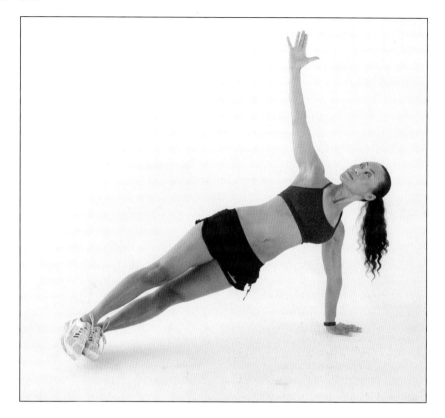

- Start by lying on your left side with your knees straight.
- Prop your upper body up on your elbow and forearm.
- Make sure that your elbow and shoulder are in line.
- Keep your abdominals and core tight and engaged.
- Raise your hips until your body forms a straight line from your ankles to your shoulders.
- Breathe deeply for the duration of the exercise.
- Hold this position for 30 seconds (or as directed). That's 1 set.
- Turn around so that you're lying on your right side and repeat.

MODIFIED SIDE PLANK

- Bend your knees 90 degrees and bring them to the floor.
- Complete the same exact motion as in the side plank, but with bent knees.
- All plank form rules apply.

FLAT ABS AND A CAST-IRON CORE

55

PLANK SWING SWITCHES

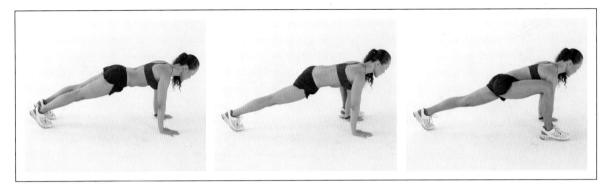

- Start off by getting into a plank position with your arms completely straight and wrists, elbows, and shoulders aligned.
- Your body should form a straight line from your head to your ankles.
- Lift one foot off the floor and jump (or step, for a modification) your leg forward and outside of your arm on the same side.
- Don't change the plank position the rest of your body is in as you move your leg.
- Ideally you should have enough mobility to bring your foot up by the arms, with a 90-degree angle in your knee.
- As you begin to jump or step the leg back, simultaneously bring up the opposite leg, stepping the foot to the hand.
- Alternate back and forth swiftly while maintaining your posture.

HALF GET-UP

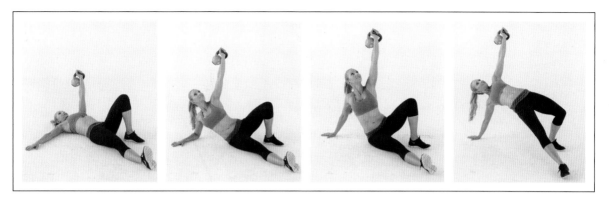

To begin, lie down with the kettlebell in your left hand and your left leg bent. Your right leg and right arm should be straight and positioned out at a 45-degree angle from your body, flat on the ground.

- Starting in the position described above, stare only at your kettlebell (never look forward or down).
- Push yourself up to your right elbow.
- Push yourself up to your right hand.
- Lift your body up by pushing your hips up to the sky.
- Pause for a second, engaging your glutes and keeping your abdominals tight.
- Continue back down through the same exact steps as when you came up. Switch sides as your workout calls for.

TURKISH SIT-UP

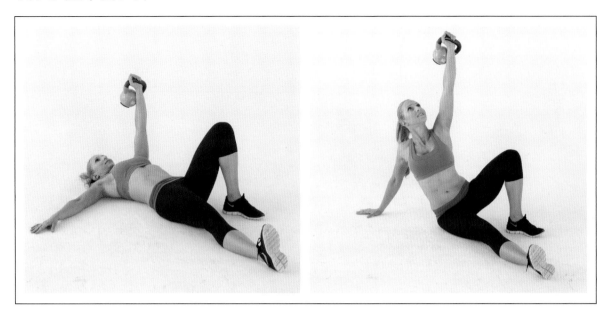

Like the half get-up, this move is similar to the Turkish get-up, which is covered on page 116.

- Start in the same position as for the half get-up, with the kettlebell overhead held by the handle in one hand. Bend the leg on the same side as the hand holding the kettlebell, while extending the other arm and leg at a 45-degree angle from your body, flat on the ground.
- Staring only at your kettlebell overhead, begin to use your abdominal strength to sit up.
- After you complete a sit-up, continue back down to the starting position. Repeat on the other side as your workout calls for.

GYMNASTICS HOLLOW

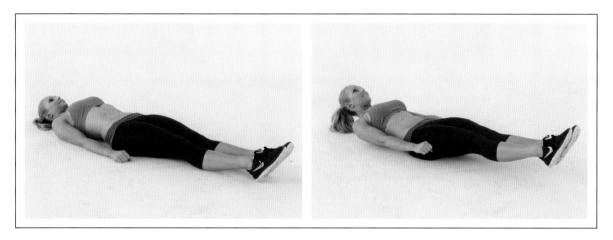

- Lie on the floor with your feet stretched out in front of you, pressing your legs together and in one straight line. Keep your hands at your hips.
- Take a moment and bring your legs up about 1 foot off of the floor as a single unit.
- Bring your arms 6 inches to 1 foot off of the floor at your sides.
- Pause, making sure everything from your shoulder blades to your tailbone is still placed on the floor.
- Then come down and repeat.

For a modification, place one foot on the ground, as pictured. Switch sides.

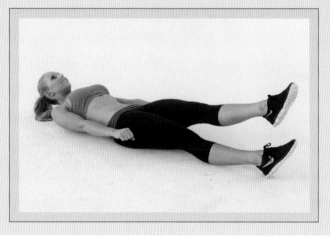

KB TWIST

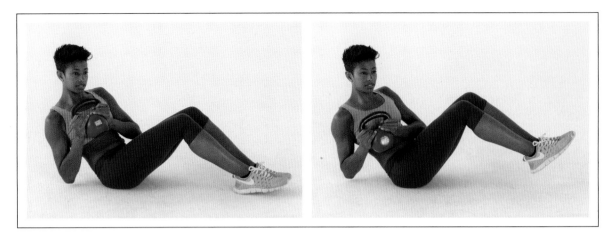

- Hold the kettlebell with both hands in a mid-racked position.
- Your shoulders should be strong and straight.
- Hold your torso at a 45-degree angle for the entire movement—your torso and the tops of your legs should make a V shape.
- Keep your feet either flat on the floor or elevated off of the floor, as shown in the advanced modification above at right, with bent knees in front of you.
- Rotate your body leading with the shoulders, not with the weight of the kettlebell.
- Do so without raising or lowering your torso.
- Go through the motion slowly and with control. Do not let the weight control your movement; instead, move through your shoulders, maintaining spinal stability the entire time.

KB CRAB REACH

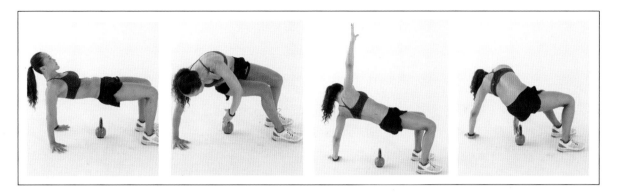

- Place the kettlebell underneath you as you post up on your hands and feet with your belly facing up.
- Engage your glutes and core.
- Take one arm off of the ground and reach around to touch the kettlebell.
- Then turn and switch sides.

KICKING CRAB REACH

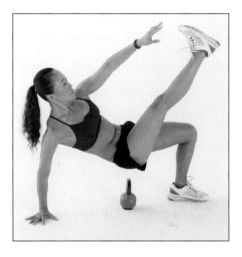

- Execute the same exact motion as above, except add in a leg kick up and reach over to touch the leg with the opposite arm.
- In both motions, make sure that there is no pressure placed on the shoulder by keeping your glutes tight the entire time.

KB KNEES

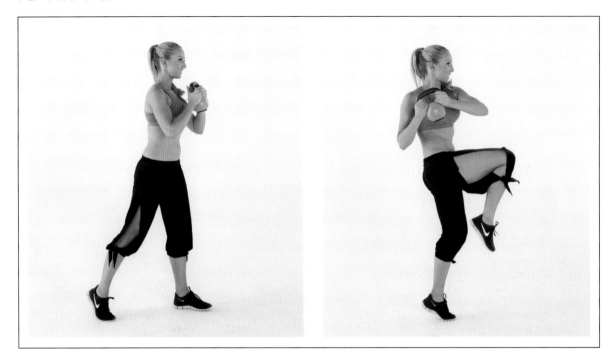

- Get into a boxing stance, left leg forward and the right leg back and out 45 degrees. Distribute the weight evenly between both legs. Bring your rear leg up on the ball of your foot so that the foot is mobile and you can pivot. This is your boxing stance.

- Keep your shoulders squared, your back straight, your hands raised by your chest, and your dominant leg just a little behind the other one at hips' width apart. With both hands, hold a kettlebell by the horns, mid-racked.

- Take your rear leg and drive it up, bending at the knee so that you are driving the crown of your knee forward and up.

- Step the knee back into your boxing stance.

- Always start the motion with the rear leg, starting from your boxing stance.

- This should feel like you are skipping.

- When you get comfortable, you can add a light hop or skip to the knee.

ALTERNATING KNEE SKIPS

For this move, do not hold a kettlebell.

- Take your rear leg and drive it up, bending at the knee so that you are driving the crown of your knee forward and up.
- As you step back, make sure that you switch the legs so that your other leg winds up being the rear leg (basically you are switching leads in your stance). This way you are alternating knees.
- Always knee with the rear leg, starting from your boxing stance.
- When you get comfortable, you can add a light hop or skip to the knee.

ALTERNATING KETTLEBELL KNEE SKIPS

- Once you are comfortable performing regular knees, you can continue to challenge yourself with the kettlebell knee.
- Hold one kettlebell in the mid-racked position, elbows tight to the body.
- Continue to get into your boxing stance, positioning your feet as illustrated, but keeping your arms tight to the body, at chest level.
- Begin to knee with the rear leg and slightly move your shoulders, not the kettlebell, to meet the knee (it should look and feel like a slight twist).
- Step back and continue to knee with the same leg, or alternate knees.

KB KNEE HOLD

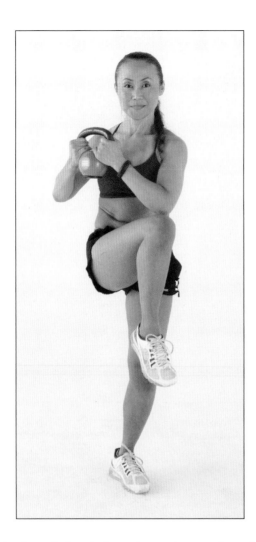

- Hold one kettlebell with both hands in the mid-racked position, elbows tight to the body.

- Get into your boxing stance, positioning your feet as illustrated earlier but keeping your arms tight to the body, at chest level.

- Begin to bring the rear leg's knee up and slightly move your shoulders, not the kettlebell, to meet the knee (it should look and feel like a slight twist).

- Now hold that position in place for 10 to 20 seconds.

- Make sure that you maintain a good posture and tight core. Do not collapse your back.

- Remember to keep your abdominals fully activated.

KNEE KICK-OUT

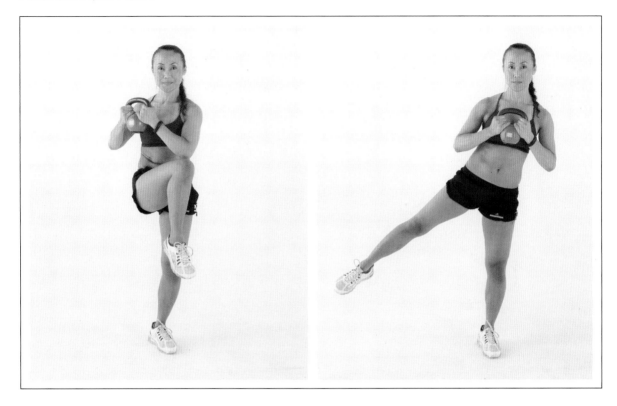

- Hold one kettlebell in mid-racked position, elbows tight to the body.
- Get into your boxing stance, but keep your arms tight to the body, at chest level.
- Bring the rear leg's knee up and slightly move your shoulders, not the kettlebell, to meet the knee (it should look and feel like a slight twist).
- Now hold that position in place for 5 to 10 seconds.
- Make sure that you maintain a good posture and tight core. Do not collapse your back.
- Remember to keep your abdominals fully activated.
- Then slowly and with full control bring the leg back—but do not step it on the floor. Instead, maintain balance and keep the leg out to the side.
- Hold for 5 to 10 seconds.
- Without stepping back down, bring the knee back up.

KB BOB AND WEAVE

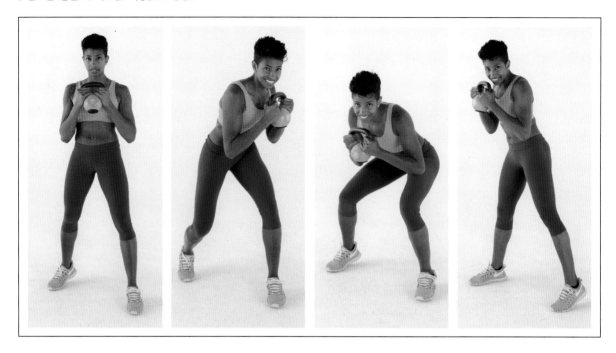

- Holding the kettlebell with both hands in a mid-racked position, take a boxing stance with one leg forward and the other behind.
- Place your weight on the ball of your rear foot and twist down a little and toward your front foot as if you are ducking a punch coming at you from your rear foot's side.
- Dip down in a mini squat and make a small half circle with your head as you come up, slightly shifting the head.
- Keep the kettlebell mid-racked, at chest level, and tight to the body.
- Switch directions, coming back through mini squat/dip to starting position.
- Do not forget to switch your stance for the next set.

DECK SQUAT

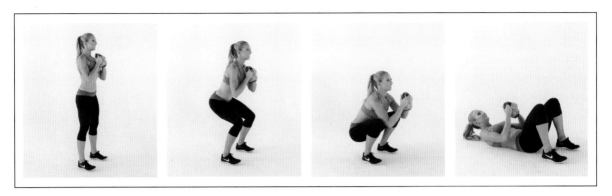

You might want to have a mat or towel to cushion your back.

- Hold the kettlebell mid-racked and tight to the chest.
- Squat down and then lie down, dropping your body in one controlled motion from standing, through a squat, all the way down to lying on your back.
- Finish the motion in a sit-up position.
- Continue back up through the sit-up and reverse squat all the way up to standing.
- Keep the kettlebell tight to the body in a mid-racked position throughout.

BONUS! Top off your deck squat with one of these four motions from other chapters in order to add a variable of strength and cardio to the mix.

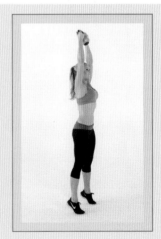

- Add a **halo** when you reach standing position
- Add a **snap or push kick** at standing position
- Add an **overhead KB press** with both arms (as pictured)
- Add a **KB knee**, or three alternating knees, at standing position

WINDMILL

We have pictured two stance options. The one with the foot facing forward is more advanced, as pictured first:

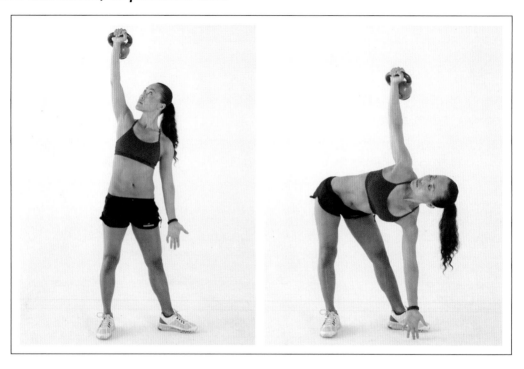

Otherwise, this is the standard move:

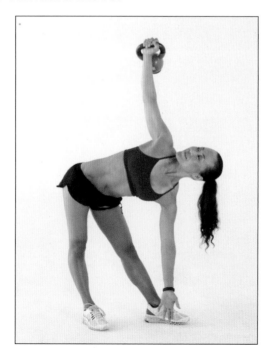

- Bring the kettlebell overhead in the racked grip with the right arm.
- Rotate both of your feet 45 degrees to the right (away from the arm).
- Keep your eyes on the kettlebell the entire time.
- Push the hip out to the left, under the supporting hand.
- Keep both knees softly straight.
- Fold at the waist and lower the torso down while keeping the kettlebell vertical overhead, with your eyes never leaving the kettlebell.
- Lower down as far as you can; it is not necessary to touch the floor.
- Extend your left arm down in front of the left leg, naturally and with the palm facing out. Switch sides as your workout calls for.

OTHER WINDMILL OPTIONS INCLUDE:
- Anchoring the lower arm with a kettlebell (but keeping an eye overhead the entire time)
- Bending the elbow of the arm that does not have a kettlebell behind the back
- Performing the same exact motion for a stretch and not holding any kettlebells

BIRD DOG

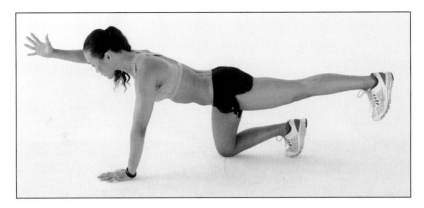

- Start out on your hands and knees.
- Make sure you keep the abdominals tight throughout the entire motion.
- Make sure that your back is strong and straight.
- Raise your right arm and left leg until they're in line with your body.
- Hold for 5 to 10 seconds and alternate sides.
- Make sure to keep your hips and lower back still, even as you switch arms and legs.

ADVANCED BIRD DOG

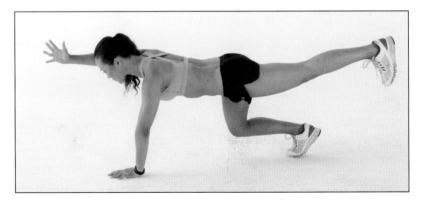

- Once you have mastered the bird dog from the knees, try it with an elevated knee.
- Bring the knee that is planted on the floor off of the ground by only 2–4 inches, keeping the knee in line with the hip.
- Hold and alternate.

THE PERFECT CORE AND ABS WORKOUT PLAN

Here are some options on how to put everything together for your workout to achieve beautiful abs and a tight core. They are in order from easiest to hardest.

For all workouts:
Start with 4–6 warm-up exercises from chapter 9.
End with 4–6 cool-down stretches from chapter 9.

Workout 1:

Complete 2 sets of any 8 exercises from this chapter.
Work with a challenging weight/pace (depending on the move) that will leave you sweating for 1 minute of work/30 seconds of rest between each set.

Workout 2:

Complete 3 sets of any 6 exercises from this chapter.
Work with a challenging weight at 8–15 reps per move.
You should feel challenged, and you should max out at the weight.

Workout 3:

Complete 4 sets of any 4 exercises from this chapter.
Work with a challenging weight/pace (depending on the move) that will leave you sweating for 1 minute of work/30 seconds of rest between each.

Workout 4:

Complete 2 sets of any 8 exercises from this chapter.
Work with a challenging weight at 8–15 reps per move.
You should feel challenged, and you should max out at the weight.

Workout 5:

Run a circuit of 8 exercises from this chapter.
Complete one full rotation of all 8 exercises: 1 minute work and 30 seconds rest.
Repeat the circuit one more time, but this time do 1 minute work and 15 seconds rest.

Workout 6:

Pick 6 exercises from this chapter and place them into the following module:

- Perform the first and second exercises you picked for 8 rounds of 20 seconds of work and 10 seconds of rest for a total of 4 minutes of work.

- Rest for 2 minutes (a more advanced routine cuts this down to 1 minute of rest).

- Perform the third and fourth exercises you picked for 8 rounds of 20 seconds of work and 10 seconds of rest for a total of 4 minutes of work.

- Rest for 2 minutes (a more advanced routine cuts this down to 1 minute of rest).

- Perform the fifth and sixth exercises you picked for 8 rounds of 20 seconds of work and 10 seconds of rest for a total of 4 minutes of work.

- Rest for 2 minutes (a more advanced routine cuts this down to 1 minute of rest).

Use the move listed or any of the move's variations:

Box A	Box B	Box C
Use any move from chapters 4, 7, or 8.	Use any move from chapter 6.	Use any move from chapter 5.

Pick 3 exercises from the boxes above; one exercise from Box A, one from Box B, and one from Box C.

Place them into the following module:

- Perform the first exercise you picked for 8 rounds of 20 seconds of work and 10 seconds of rest for a total of 4 minutes of work.
- Rest for 2 minutes (a more advanced routine cuts this down to 1 minute of rest).
- Perform the second exercise you picked for 8 rounds of 20 seconds of work and 10 seconds of rest for a total of 4 minutes of work.
- Rest for 2 minutes (a more advanced routine cuts this down to 1 minute of rest).
- Perform the third exercise you picked for 8 rounds of 20 seconds of work and 10 seconds of rest for a total of 4 minutes of work.
- Rest for 2 minutes (a more advanced routine cuts this down to 1 minute of rest).
- Stretch using 3–6 stretches from chapter 9.

CHAPTER 6

ULTIMATE ARMS AND BACK

Prevent Shoulder Injury and Sculpt an Amazing Upper Body

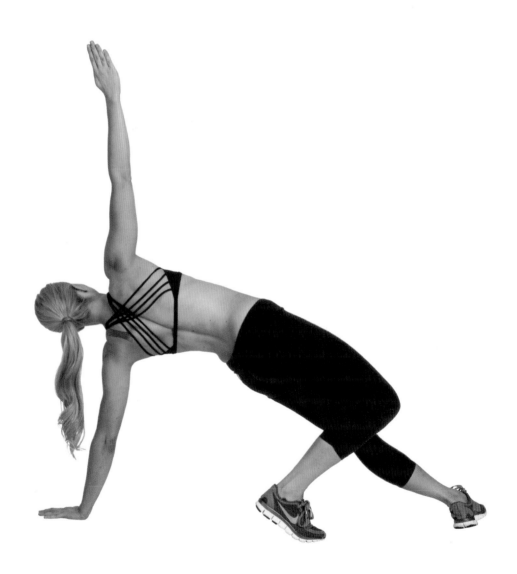

You can't always flaunt your toned legs, emphasize great glutes, or bare a firm midsection. However, the arms are one area of the body that can be shown off in almost every season and every outfit. The back is another area of the body that can showcase all of the hard work and dedication you have placed into your training regimen. If we look at your upper body, strong and defined arms and a great back, chest, and shoulders can make your waist look slimmer, as well as help you function more efficiently in your daily chores and your recreational sport activities. It's not just athletes who need upper body strength to throw, catch, punch, push, or pull; everyone can benefit from spend most of the day strength, including women who carry their kids, walk their dogs, carry groceries, and even move their own furniture (just to give a few examples). In reality, everyone could benefit from a stronger upper body.

Our sedentary lifestyles in which we spend most of the day sitting don't just create issues in the lower part of the body. Poor posture can affect the length tension relationships in your back, causing neck and back pain, headaches, a forward neck tilt, and collapsed shoulders. Not only is this bad aesthetically, but it can also cause weaknesses that create pain and major imbalances, which can lead to shoulder, neck, and back injuries during times we are active. It is for all of these reasons that the upper body should be strengthened evenly, incorporating vertical and horizontal pushing and pulling motions, as well as spine activation and postural corrective exercises.

Basically, your upper body is not just a bicep or a tricep. You have major muscles that are itching to get activated! It's important for you to understand that the health of your body depends on activating them evenly and equally in a variety of movements.

Another major reason to strengthen the arms? Your shoulder has the greatest range of motion in the entire body; therefore, if the upper body is weak, your shoulder is far more susceptible to injury (both overuse and acute injury). It is for this reason that you should have a balanced and healthy strength training routine that includes every area of the body.

I've never heard anyone complain of a bulky back, and there's a reason for this. Your back muscles are beautiful, and the more you train them, the more you will see a change in your body composition (including the belly and legs!). Since muscle needs more energy to function than fat does, the amazing and functional muscles you build in your upper body will help you burn fat from your midsection and legs. That's a fact!

UPPER BODY ANATOMY

ARMS

Biceps are the muscles in the upper front of your arms. These guys help in bending the elbow, like in a bicep curl, and rotating the forearm.

Forearms include the flexors of the fingers (those bend the wrist forward) and the extensors in your wrists (they bend the wrists back).

Triceps are the muscles in the upper back of your arms. Their main job is to help you straighten your arm.

BACK

Your back muscles include:

Latissimus dorsi: one of the largest muscles in the back. It helps with pulling and grabbing motions by helping the arms extend, rotate, and adduct.

Trapezius: the muscle that lets you shrug your shoulders.

Rhomboids: rhombus-shaped muscles responsible for pulling your shoulder blades together, along with the traps.

SHOULDERS

The **deltoid** muscle of the shoulder has three areas: the middle, anterior, and posterior delt. The **posterior deltoid** is used to pull your arm backward.

Rotator cuff: has a series of muscles that work to stabilize your shoulder and are worked in a great variety of upper body motions.

Serratus anterior: helps stabilize and rotate the shoulder blade.

Levator scapulae: this muscle is important because it really runs along the back of your neck, attaches into the shoulder, and helps with motions like stabilizing the neck and shrugging the shoulders.

CHEST

Pectoralis major: pulls the arms toward the middle of the body.

Pectoralis minor: helps to pull the shoulders forward.

Okay! Now that we met the muscles, let's train them. The most important things we can say about **kettlebells and your upper body** are right here:

- Despite what it looks like, **the kettlebell swing does not work the arms**! No matter how beautiful you want your arms to look, resist the urge to lift the kettlebell with your arms when swinging. The kettlebell swing is a posterior chain motion, and should only work the back muscles and a little of the anterior deltoids. But all of the power in a correct kettlebell swing is generated with your hips, specifically your gluteal muscles, not your arms.

- Kettlebells give us countless option to train the chest, arms, upper body, shoulders, and back. Exercises include a bottoms-up press, true high-pulls, and halos.

- **If you push, you must pull!** Remember that the body has to be a yin-yang of balance. If you push, you must include a pull in your exercises routine, either in the same day or in the same week. Examples of Kettlebell Kickboxing pulls are leopard pulls and rows, while examples of pushes are push-ups and presses.

- The shoulder is one of the most common points of injury—so be careful! When you begin to lose your form, it is time to stop that move, check your form, rest, or change to a lighter kettlebell weight. Remember that you should never injure yourself during exercise!

YOUR EXERCISES!

HIGH PULLS

A kettlebell high pull starts with a traditional kettlebell swing before changing into a pull at the top, so yes—you will be getting amazing glutes, core, and leg action just as you do for swings. However, the actual pull at the top of the motion turn this into an amazing back and shoulder motion for your upper body. Another bonus—because of all of the muscles you are using, this motion is huge on calorie burn! Make sure to follow the basic traditional swing form covered in chapter 4.

RECAP: Basic Swing Form

- Pick up the kettlebell by the handle and sit back, bending first at the hips, and then at the knees in a hinge.
- As you hinge and swing the kettlebell back and behind the knees, thrust your hips forward and raise your torso back to the standing position, then continue without stopping back down into your hinge.
- Create a nonstop fluid motion of the swing; the kettlebell going behind the knees and back up to shoulder level.
- Do not raise the kettlebell with your arms. Your arms are weightless, as is the kettlebell, through the entire motion.
- Squeeze your glutes as you push your hips forward, making sure your butt muscles are engaged and working.
- Squeeze your glutes tight and do not backward bend at the top of the motion.
- At the top of the swing, remember to keep your arms straight, thrust your hips forward, straighten your knees, and swing the kettlebell no higher than chest level as you rise to a standing position and engage the glutes (squeeze the butt muscles together).

MAKE IT A SINGLE-ARM HIGH PULL

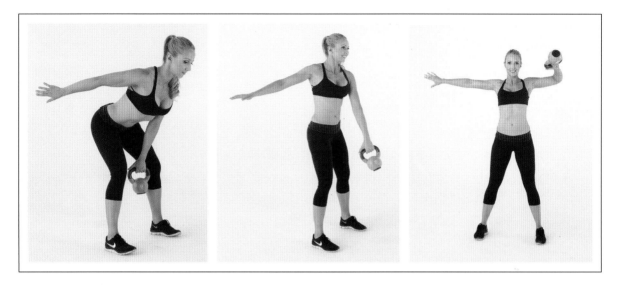

- You will be swinging the kettlebell with either your left or right arm.
- When you swing the kettlebell with one arm, make sure that as the kettlebell travels back and behind the legs, your thumb faces back, not forward. This helps protect the elbow from hyperextension.
- Shoulder stability becomes more important with one arm. Keep your shoulder engaged, with the shoulder blade tucked in and fixed.
- As the kettlebell begins to come up, **high pull** it to one side (see the third photo above).
- As you pull, your stance and the hip-thrusting motion never change from the traditional kettlebell swing.
- At the top of the pull, your kettlebell should wind up lined up with, or slightly higher than, the shoulder and elbow at a 90-degree angle at the side you are pulling toward.
- It is really important to engage the lats to prevent the shoulders from twisting.
- Think of the arm as a cable, merely holding the kettlebell with no tension.
- Do not try to lift the kettlebell with the muscles of the arm. Remember that this is a motion that engages your glutes and posterior chain, not the arms or quads.
- This is a single-side, single-arm high pull, so stick to one side for the desired number or reps or time.

MAKE IT A SWITCHING HIGH PULL

- As you complete the high pull on one side, swing the kettlebell back down and then up and perform a kettlebell swing switch to the other arm.
- When you switch the kettlebell, turn your palm up to hand over the kettlebell, making sure you are hinging and engaging the posterior chain at the top of the kettlebell exchange, just like at the top of a regular kettlebell swing.
- Make sure to swing the kettlebell back down after the swing switch.
- Only then can you come up for a high pull on the other side.
- Continue to alternate.

MAKE IT A DOUBLE-ARM HIGH PULL

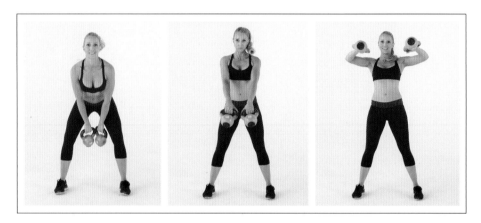

- Perform the exact same motion as illustrated in the single-arm high pull, except you will work with double kettlebells.
- Pull the kettlebells up simultaneously.

MAKE IT A LADDER HIGH PULL

A ladder high pull starts with single-arm high pulls, one on each side with a switch between, and then increases to two reps on each side with a switch between, and so on, adding one rep on each side between the switches. This continues to build as you build a ladder to more reps on each side.

- Start off with one high pull on your left, and then switch and perform on the other side.
- On your next set, perform two high pulls on the left, and then switch and perform two high pulls on the right.
- Continue to build your numbers of high pulls on each side.

SNATCH

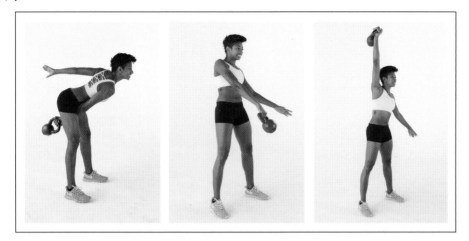

- Perform the single-arm high pull from the swing to the top of the high pull.
- At the top of the high pull, open the hand wide and continue the upward movement of the kettlebell by thrusting the hand through the handle toward the ceiling.
- As you exhale, straighten the elbow and pause for a moment with your leg, elbow, shoulder, and wrist in a straight line, holding the kettlebell overhead.
- Bend your arm slightly and allow the kettlebell to free-fall down between the legs.
- It is important not to allow the kettlebell to go too far down; at the bottom of the movement, keep the wrist at pubic bone level.
- Remember that the kettlebell is snatched overhead using the posterior chain, not the arm.

KB CATCH SWING TO LIFT

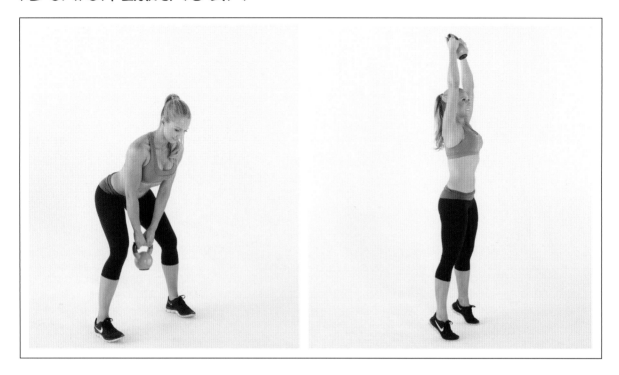

- The foundation of this motion is the kettlebell swing, followed by the kettlebell squat.
- Hold the kettlebell with both hands.
- Start a traditional kettlebell swing, but break the swing the moment the kettlebell begins to come past your knees on the way up. Pull the kettlebell straight up to your chest instead of finishing the swing.
- As you break the swing, bend your arms at the elbows and catch the kettlebell, placing it into a mid-racked position at your chest. (All swing motions and fundamentals still apply—this is still a hinge position.)
- Hold the kettlebell fixed and steady in mid-racked position.
- Press the kettlebell overhead until both arms are completely straight. Pause for just a moment at the top.
- When finished, bring the kettlebell back down to mid-racked position and then slide it back down to change the grip from mid-racked to a hanging bell.
- At the same time, hinge back into the swing.
- Swing the kettlebell back, and again break it halfway on the way up and continue the motion.
- Make sure to squeeze your glutes at the top of the kettlebell catch, just as you would in your kettlebell swing.

BOTTOMS-UP LIFT/TRUE HIGH PULL

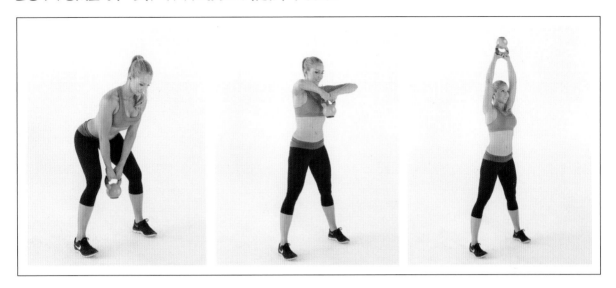

- Begin in a swing stance, with the kettlebell hanging down and your shoulders and back straight.
- Make sure your hips sit back farther than your knees (you are not squatting).
- Instead of swinging the bell, you will be using a rectilinear motion (not curvilinear like in a swing).
- Dip down a little bit into your hinge, engaging the glutes and using that momentum begin to lift the kettlebell straight up (do not swing it).
- As you lift the kettlebell up, note you are going strictly up; do not extend the kettlebell in front of you.
- As you begin to lift the bell up to chest level, begin to turn over the kettlebell into a bottoms-up position and continue to bring the kettlebell overhead until your arms are fully extended overhead.
- Do not pause.
- Begin to bring the kettlebell back down the same way. Do not extend the kettlebell in front of you; instead, drop it directly down, and turn it from a bottoms-up to a hanging position immediately after you pass chest level.
- Repeat in a steady and continuous form.

PUSH-UP

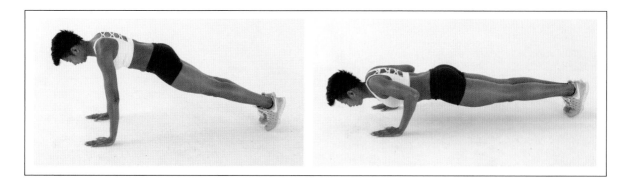

- Starting in a plank position, get down on all fours and place your hands on the floor so that they're in line with your elbows and shoulders. Straighten your legs out behind you, with your weight on your toes.
- Your elbows, shoulders, and wrists should be in line.
- Squeeze your glutes and hold them that way for the entire movement. Keep your core tight, like in a plank.
- Try to keep your hips in line with your upper body and do not allow your back to sink in—stay in a straight plank.
- Your body should form a straight line from your ankles to your head, abdominals tight.
- Your arms should be straight when starting.
- As you lower your body to the ground, make sure not to overflare your elbows.
- As you lower your body, make sure your elbows come outward and back toward your knees at the same time—the bend should be out and half back.
- Lower your body until your chest nearly touches the floor.
- Tuck your elbows as you lower your body so that your upper arms form a 45-degree angle with your body in the bottom position of the movement.
- Pause at the bottom and then push yourself back to the starting position as quickly as possible.

Form

- Do not let hips or back sag at any point during the exercise; this means that your form has broken down.
- Make sure that you do not feel any pain in your shoulders—a push-up should not hurt your shoulder joint.
- If you feel any of this, consider that your last repetition and end the set.

MODIFIED PUSH-UP

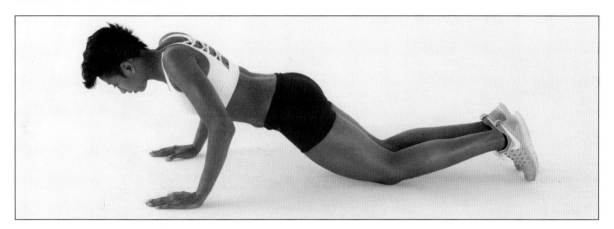

- Execute the same motion as previously illustrated, but with your knees bent and on the floor (to take some of the weight off of the push-up).

> In a modified push-up, you are still using more than 50 percent of your bodyweight.

SEMI-MODIFIED PUSH-UP

- Execute the same motion as in the modified push-up, but bend your knees on the way up (lower down in a regular push-up and come up on a modified push-up).

NEGATIVE PUSH-UP

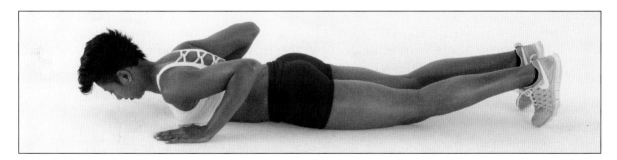

- Execute the same motion as the push-up, just lower yourself all the way down to the ground until you are laying on the ground fully relaxed.
- Then engage the abdominal muscles, glutes, and back and bring yourself back up to plank.

ADVANCED PUSH-UP VERSIONS

Kettlebell Push-Up

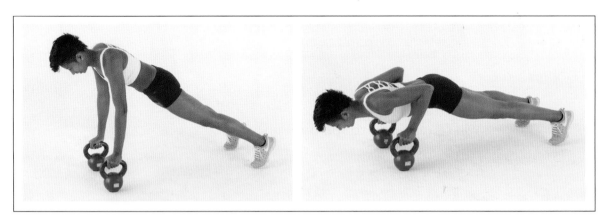

- Execute the push-up while elevated on two kettlebells.
- Grip the kettlebell handles and make sure to open your legs up into a wider stance than your regular push-up for balance.
- Keep your core tight.
- Note that this is a very advanced motion.

3-Way Push-Up

- Do a standard push-up, but pause for three seconds at three points of the push-up.
- Pause halfway down, pause at the very bottom, and then pause at the halfway point on the way back up.

This push-up will also help build negative and isometric (or stationary) strength, thus affecting your positive strength.

30-30-30 Push-Up

- Take 30 full seconds to lower down.
- Take 30 full seconds to come up.
- Take 30 full seconds to come back down.
- Follow full push-up form as seen in the regular push-up.
- If this is too difficult, try a modified version (with bent knees).

KB FIRE DRILL

- Start standing, then either step or jump back into plank position.
- Perform a negative push-up, laying the body all the way down to the ground.
- Then roll the body over and post back up from lying flat on the belly to a plank.
- Continue by lowering yourself down to the ground again and rolling back to starting position.
- The drill will require you to roll back and forth.

KB FIRE DRILL KICKER

- Complete the fire drill motion exactly as described above, except that when you roll over and get into a plank, continue to stand all the way up with either a jump up or a step up.
- Then as you are standing, perform a snap kick.
- Following your snap kick, lower back down and continue to perform the fire drill.

SPIDERMAN PUSH-UP

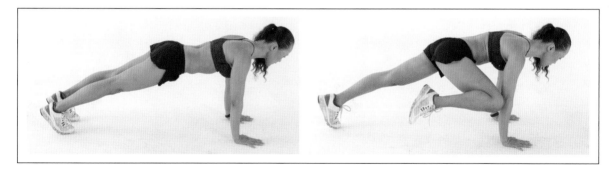

- Start in a plank position.
- Follow all standard forms of the basic push-up.
- Lift your right foot off the floor and try to touch your knee to your elbow.
- Bring your foot back to standard push-up position and continue to execute a regular or modified push-up.
- Make sure to alternate left and right.

ADVANCED SPIDERMAN

- Start in a plank position.
- Lift your right foot off the floor and try to touch your knee to your elbow as you lower down to the push-up.
- Reverse the movement, then push your body back to the starting position. Repeat on your next repetition, touching your left knee to your left elbow.
- Make sure to alternate left and right.

SPIDER SWITCHES TO PUSH-UPS

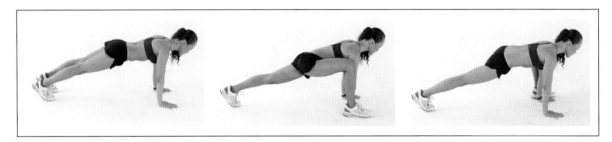

- Start in a plank position.
- Follow all standard forms of the basic push-up.
- Then, after one push-up, lift your right foot off the floor and jump (advanced) or step (modified) the foot up to your hands and align the foot and both arms (as pictured).
- Immediately jump your foot back as you switch and bring the opposite foot up to the hands.
- Complete two rotations of this and then continue to do a push-up (regular or modified).
- Then do two more rotations of jumping and switching the legs again, and then a push-up.

LEOPARD PUSH-UP

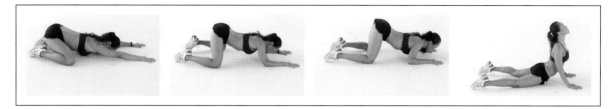

- Begin in a child's pose, with your arms stretched out in front of you and your hips sitting back on your knees.

- From there, begin to pull your body forward like a wave until your nose nearly touches the floor.

- Lower your hips until they almost touch the floor, as you simultaneously raise your head and shoulders toward the ceiling.

- Engage your back, abdominals, and glutes. Do not flare the elbows, and make sure your back is working.

- When finished, get back to a child's pose and start over again.

ADVANCED:
Reverse the movement back to the starting position the same way you came into the position.

FULL LEOPARD PUSH-UP

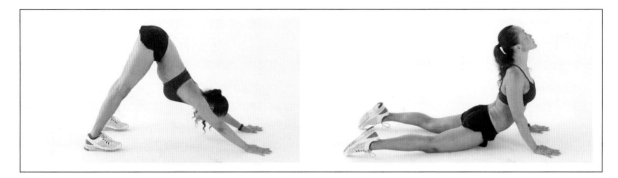

- Begin in standard push-up position, then shift your body up into a downward dog position (an upside-down V).
- In a downward dog position, your hips should be shooting up to the ceiling, and your arms and legs should have equal amount of weight distribution.
- Keeping your hips elevated, lower your body from chest to hips, like a wave, until your nose nearly touches the floor.
- Lower your hips until they almost touch the floor, as you simultaneously raise your head and shoulders toward the ceiling.
- Engage your back, abdominals, and glutes. Do not flare the elbows and make sure your back is working.
- When finished, get back to a plank and start over again.

ADVANCED:
Reverse the movement back to the starting position the same way you came into the position.

LEOPARD BURPEES

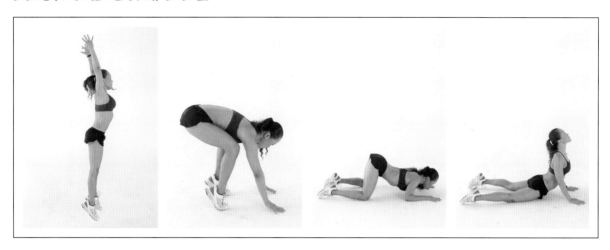

- Start in standing position and push off the floor into a vertical jump, using your glutes and legs to jump.
- For a modified version, just reach up, without jumping.
- Continue down to the floor through a forward bend. Then jump back into a plank.
- From the plank, sit back into child's pose.
- From there, begin to pull your body forward like a wave until your nose nearly touches the floor.
- Lower your hips until they almost touch the floor, as you simultaneously raise your head and shoulders toward the ceiling.
- Engage your back, abdominals, and glutes. Do not flare the elbows and make sure your back is working.
- When finished, get back to child's pose and jump back up to standing. Repeat.

ADVANCED:
Do the entire motion with a full leopard push-up.

KETTLEBELL ROW

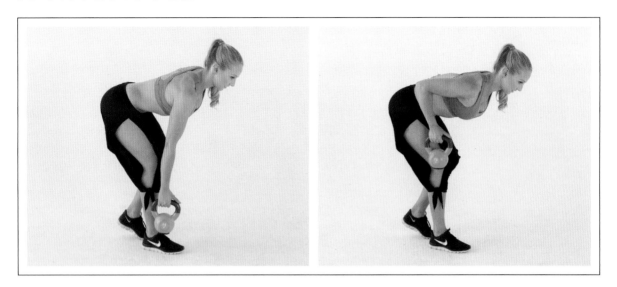

- Grab a kettlebell in your right hand. Bend at your hips and knees (in a full hinge, **not** a squat).
- Lower your torso until it's almost parallel to the floor and your back is completely straight.
- Your neck should be aligned with your body, in line with the hips.
- Let the kettlebell hang at arm's length from your shoulder, but make sure your shoulder is packed into the body, not just hanging down.
- Keep your core super tight and engaged.
- Use a neutral kettlebell grip, so that your thumb is facing forward, not out.
- Keep the elbow tight to the body.
- Pull the kettlebell to the side of your torso.
- Do not turn, rotate, or lift your torso as you row the weight up.
- Aim to use your back, not your arms.
- At the bottom, the arm should be completely extended without the kettlebell touching the ground.

DOUBLE ALTERNATING KETTLEBELL ROW

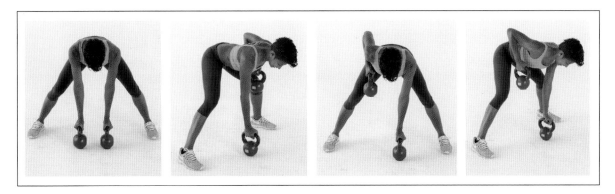

- You will need two kettlebells.
- Perform one kettlebell row with one arm, and then repeat on the other side.

DOUBLE KETTLEBELL ROW

- You will need two kettlebells.
- Row both kettlebells at the same time.

KB PUSH-UP AND ROW

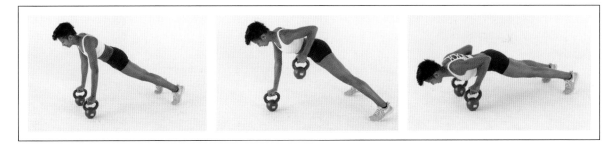

- You will need an equally weighted pair of kettlebells.
- Place them where you would traditionally position your hands in a push-up.
- Grasp the kettlebell handles and set yourself in push-up position.
- Engage your core! Pay attention to your form; this is an advanced motion.
- Set your feet wide, in a triangle, for balance.
- Note that the standard plank form is far more advanced.
- Lower your body to the floor, pause, then push yourself back up, as you would in a push-up.
- Once you're back in the starting position, row the kettlebell on one side by pulling it upward and bending your arm.

- Do not twist or rotate your body.
- Lower the kettlebell back down with control, and then repeat the same movement with your other arm.

KB FLOOR CHEST PRESS

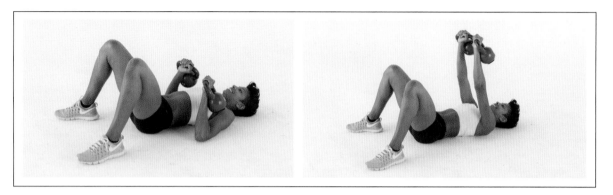

- You will need an equally weighted pair of kettlebells. Place one on each side of your mat and lie in the middle.
- Pick them up, one at a time, by the handle, weaving your hand into the handle until it's hooked in, in racked position.
- Lie faceup on the floor, abdominals and core engaged. Your knees should be bent.
- Hold the kettlebells above your chest with your arms straight.
- Lower the kettlebells until your upper arms touch the floor.
- Continue to press the weights back up to the starting position.

ALTERNATING KB FLOOR CHEST PRESS

- Follow the same exact motions as for the floor chest press, but instead of pressing both kettlebells up at the same time, alternate each one.

ALTERNATING STATIC KB FLOOR CHEST PRESS

- Follow the same exact motions as for the floor chest press.
- Bring one kettlebell up above the head and hold it there, making sure it is securely situated above the head.
- Continue to press the other kettlebell up overhead and back down, all while holding the other kettlebell overhead.
- After you complete one rep, bring that kettlebell up and hold it overhead as you complete a rep with the opposite side.

KB PRESS

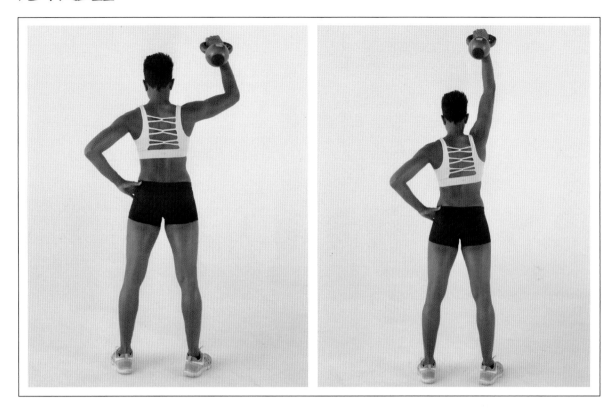

- Start out holding a kettlebell in a racked position.
- Keep your core engaged.
- Your feet should be shoulders' width apart, and your knees slightly bent.
- Press the kettlebell directly above your shoulders until your arm is completely straight.
- Slowly lower the kettlebell back to the starting position.

Make sure to take advantage of your negative reps! When you lower a kettlebell or any weight down in a press, you should engage your back and lower slowly, feeling the motion in your arms, back, and shoulders. Negative reps help build positive strength, and engaging the muscles burns bonus calories and helps you build lean muscle!

DOUBLE KB PRESS

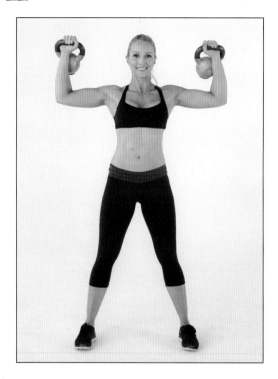

- Start out holding two kettlebells in a racked position.
- Keep your core engaged.
- Your feet should be shoulders' width apart, and your knees slightly bent.
- Press both kettlebells directly above your shoulders until your arms are completely straight.
- Slowly lower the kettlebells back to the starting position.
- Don't forget to maximize the negative rep!

ALTERNATING KB PRESS

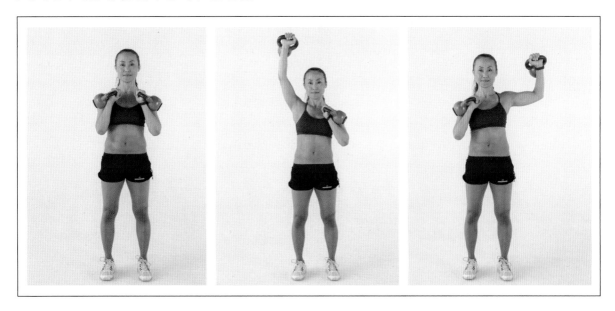

- Start out holding two kettlebell in a racked position.
- Keep your core engaged.
- Your feet should be shoulders' width apart, and your knees slightly bent.
- Press one kettlebell directly above your shoulders until your arms are completely straight.
- Slowly lower the kettlebell back to the starting position.
- Don't forget to maximize the negative rep!
- Then continue on to the other arm, alternating the presses.

RECIPROCAL KB PRESSES

- Start out holding two kettlebells in a racked position.

- Keep your core engaged.

- Your feet should be shoulders' width apart, and your knees slightly bent.

- Press one kettlebell directly above your shoulders until your arms are completely straight.

- Slowly lower one kettlebell back to the starting position as you lift the other kettlebell up—making the up/down motions overlap.

- Don't forget to maximize the negative reps!

MID-BACK KB PRESS

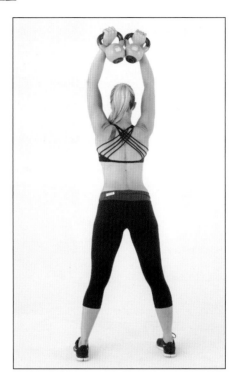

- Start out holding two kettlebells in a racked position.
- Keep your core engaged.
- Your feet should be shoulders' width apart, and your knees slightly bent.
- Press both kettlebells directly above your shoulders until your arms are straight. Curve the kettlebells in slightly so that the belly of the bells touch each other at the top, engaging the mid-back.
- Slowly lower the kettlebells back to the starting position.
- Don't forget to maximize the negative rep!

PUSH PRESS

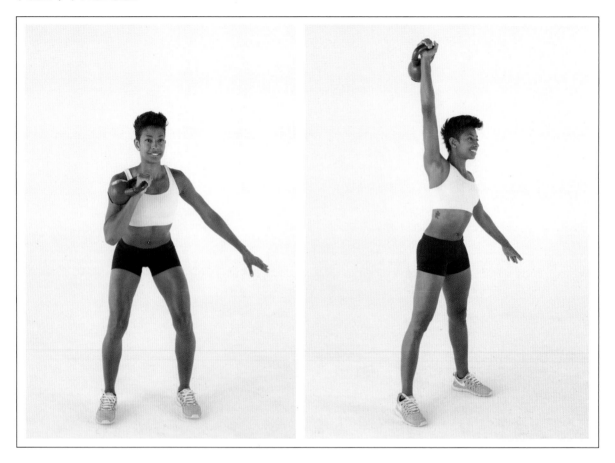

- Start out holding a kettlebell in a racked position.

- Keep your core engaged.

- Your feet should be shoulders' width apart.

- Bend your knees to a quarter squat, just enough to help you generate more power to press the kettlebell.

- You will be using the push from a semi-squatting motion to help you get the kettlebell up into a full extension overhead.

- Make sure that you explosively push up with your legs and glutes as you press the kettlebell over your head.

DOUBLE KB PUSH PRESS

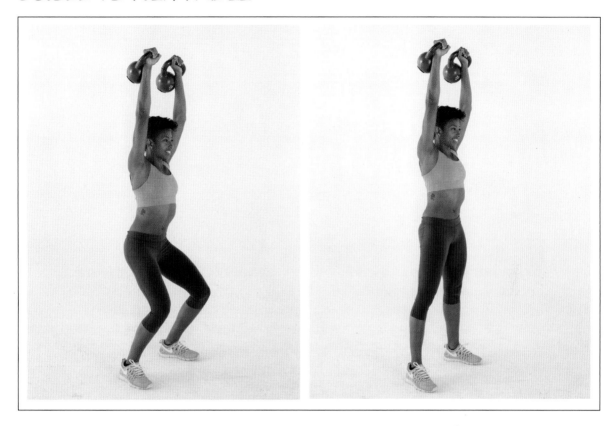

- Start out holding two kettlebells in a racked position.
- Execute the same exact motion as the single push press just discussed, except push-press two kettlebells at the same time.

SINGLE-ARM KB CLEAN

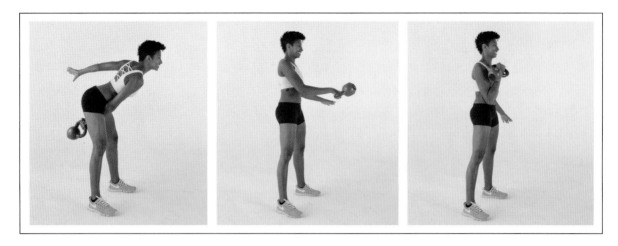

The clean is a fundamental kettlebell motion that often serves as a transition to other motions. When you clean the kettlebell, you are swinging the kettlebell back using the form of a kettlebell swing, but you will be breaking the motion the moment the kettlebell begins to come up from behind the legs. As the motion "breaks," you are going to corkscrew or rotate the kettlebell up to a racked position at your chest.

- Hold the kettlebell in a single-arm swing position.
- The thumb should be facing the body (facing down/back, not facing up).
- You will use a mini swing (the traditional swing form applies—remember to hinge!).
- Start the mini swing, but break the motion of the full swing and rotate the kettlebell around the forearm as you bring it up to racked position at your chest.
- At the top, the upper arm should be tight to the rib cage.
- The kettlebell should be resting firmly and easily between the upper arm, forearm, and shoulder against the body (not out in any way).
- The racked position of the bell should feel comfortable and natural; you should not be straining wrists or elbows, and the kettlebell should feel like it is resting on your forearm.
- With a slight lift at the elbow, the kettlebell will drop between the legs as the hips move back in a hinge and you continue to the next rep of your clean.
- Make sure to squeeze your glutes at the top of the clean, just like you would in your kettlebell swing.

DOUBLE KETTLEBELL CLEAN

- Use the same exact motion and technique as the single-arm clean; however, you will do this with two kettlebells.

- You might need to take a slightly wider stance (depending on kettlebell size).

- Please note that everything for the double kettlebell clean will remain the same as in the single-arm clean, including facing your thumbs back toward the body, not up, when you swing back.

KB CLEAN AND PRESS

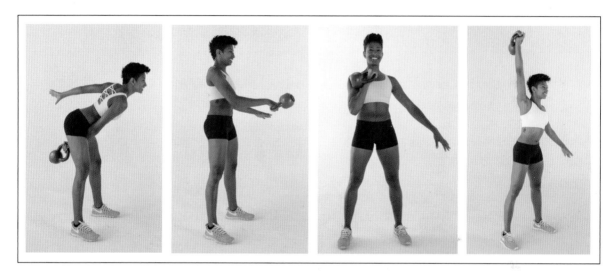

- Use the exact same motion as described in the clean.

- Once the kettlebell is in a racked position, instead of bringing it back down, continue to press the kettlebell up overhead.

- Use the same exact form as illustrated in the press step-by-step instructions.

- Continue down from the press to racked position; from this position continue right back down to perform your next set of a clean to press.

Form

- Do not curl up the kettlebell. Remember it's not a curl; it's a clean.

- Do not bang your wrist with the kettlebell; the motion must be seamless.

DOUBLE KB CLEAN AND PRESS

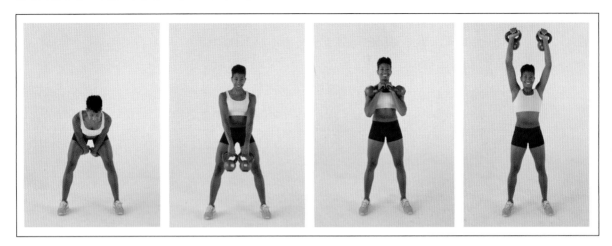

- Use the exact same motion as described in the double kettlebell clean.
- Once the kettlebells are in a racked position, instead of bringing them back down, continue to press the kettlebells up overhead.
- Use the same exact form as illustrated in the double kettlebell press step-by-step instructions.
- Continue down from the press to racked position, and from the racked position continue right back down to perform your next set of a clean to press.

DOUBLE KB CLEAN AND PUSH PRESS

- Use the exact same motion as described in the double kettlebell clean.
- Once the kettlebells are in a racked position, instead of bringing them back down, continue to push-press the kettlebells up overhead.
- Use the same exact form as illustrated in the double kettlebell push press step-by-step instructions, pushing off with a mini squat to help press the kettlebell directly overhead.
- Continue down from the press to racked position, and from the racked position continue right back down to perform your next set of a clean to push press.

KB JERK

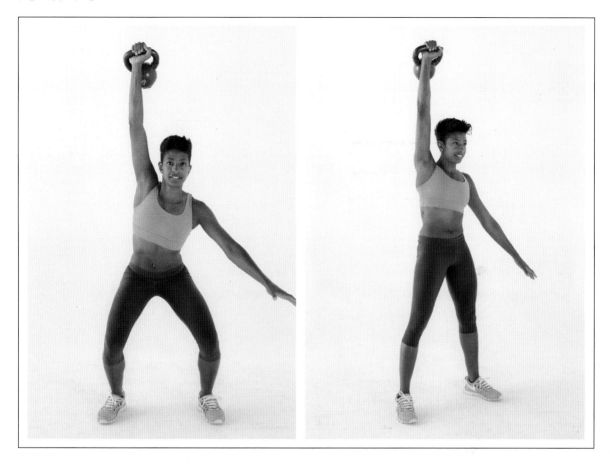

- Rack up a kettlebell.
- Dip your knees.
- Explosively push up with your legs as you press the kettlebell over your head.
- As you press the kettlebell, split your legs apart so that you land in a staggered stance, one foot in front of the other, and give a final push to the kettlebell as it goes overhead.

ADVANCED:
The same move can be done with double kettlebells.

KB CURL

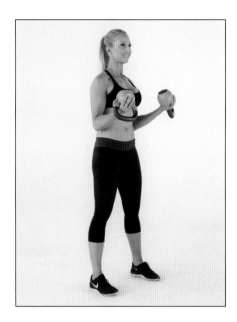

- Grab a pair of kettlebells, but instead of holding them by the handle, take them by the belly of the bell.
- Grip the kettlebells, one in each arm, by the body of the bell, looping your hand through the handle.
- Turn your arms so that your palms face upward.
- Set your feet shoulders' width apart, with a slight knee bend.
- Bend your elbows and curl the kettlebells as close to your shoulders as you can.
- Don't move your entire arm; just move the arm below the elbow.
- Don't swing into the motion; make sure you are using your arms only, no momentum.
- Pause at the top for a second, and then slowly lower the weights back to the starting position.
- Straighten your arms and repeat.

Don't neglect the negative motion. Remember that negative strength helps build positive strength, so make sure you are lowering the kettlebells slowly and effectively.

Note: You can also single-arm curl.

ALTERNATING CURL

- Alternate the curls using the form just illustrated.
- Make sure you complete one full curl before you start the next one.

RECIPROCAL CURLS

- You will need two kettlebells.
- Perform the same exact curl as illustrated in the basic kettlebell curl, but your timing on the curl will change.
- Slowly lower one kettlebell back to the starting position as you lift the other kettlebell up—making the up/down motions overlap.
- Don't forget to maximize the negative reps!

HAMMER KB CURLS

- Perform the same kettlebell curl as illustrated, except for your starting grip.
- When you start, have the same grip on the kettlebell, but instead of facing your palms upward, turn them to face your legs—inward.
- Then continue on to the same form as in your original kettlebell curl.
- This can be executed with a single kettlebell or with doubles; alternating, reciprocal, or at the same time.

STATIC HOLD KETTLEBELL CURL

- You will need two kettlebells.
- Execute the kettlebell curl.
- When you bring up one kettlebell and perform a full curl, bring the same kettlebell back halfway.
- Hold the kettlebell halfway at a 90-degree angle, making sure the elbow is close to the body.
- While you hold the kettlebell at 90 degrees, curl the other kettlebell in one full set.
- Then bring that kettlebell back to 90 degrees as you curl the other kettlebell in a full rep.

KB CURL AND PRESS

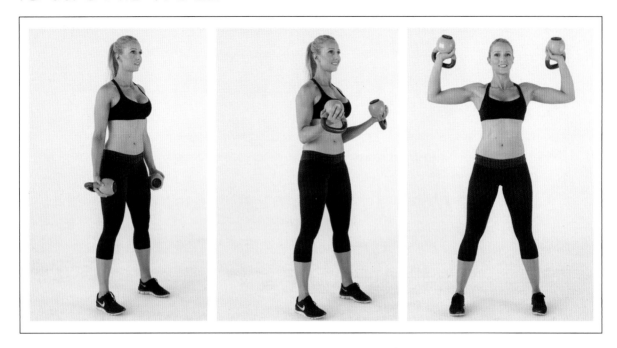

- Have two kettlebells extended down at your sides, your palms facing up.
- Make sure to have the same grip as we illustrated in the kettlebell curl, hands gripping the belly of the bell.
- Curl the kettlebells up, but do not lower down.
- Press the kettlebells above your head until your arms are straight, using the form illustrated in the press step-by-step instructions.
- Bring the kettlebells all the way back down from the negative press to the negative curl.

DOUBLE-ARM KB CURL

- With one kettlebell, start in a mid-racked position (kettlebell at chest level, gripped by the horns by both hands).
- Stand up straight, keeping your core strong and tight, with your feet shoulders' width apart.
- Slowly lower the kettlebell down to arm's length.
- Then bend the arms back up in a curl.

OVERHEAD TRICEP KETTLEBELL EXTENSION

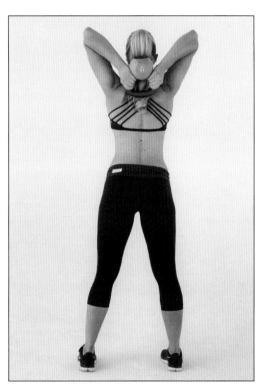

- With one kettlebell, start in a mid-racked position (kettlebell at chest level, gripped by the horns by both hands).
- Stand up straight, keeping your core strong and tight, with your feet shoulders' width apart.
- Bring your arms up and overhead to a full extension, holding the kettlebell.
- Without moving your upper arms, simply bend your elbows to lower the kettlebell behind you.
- Then slowly return back to mid-racked position.

HALO

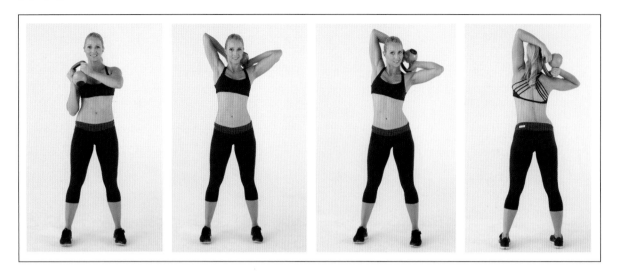

- Start off gripping the kettlebell by the horns.
- Options include having the base of the bell up or down.
- Begin to rotate the kettlebell around the head.
- Make sure to keep the kettlebell close to the head throughout the full rotation.
- Make sure the kettlebell is not over the head, but rotates directly around the head.
- You can alternate sides, work for a specific number of reps per side, or work to rotate to one side for a specific time interval before changing to rotate to the other side.

KB FARMER'S CARRY

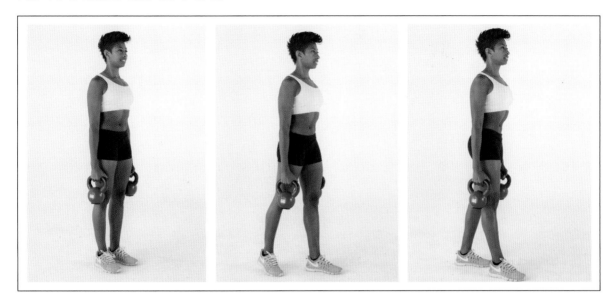

- You will need a pair of kettlebells that are of challenging weight.
- Let them hang naturally, at arm's length, next to your sides, with a grip such that the thumbs are facing forward.
- The farmer's carry is just a walk holding the kettlebells.
- If you can walk for longer than one minute, you should try a heavier weight.

JAB-CROSS

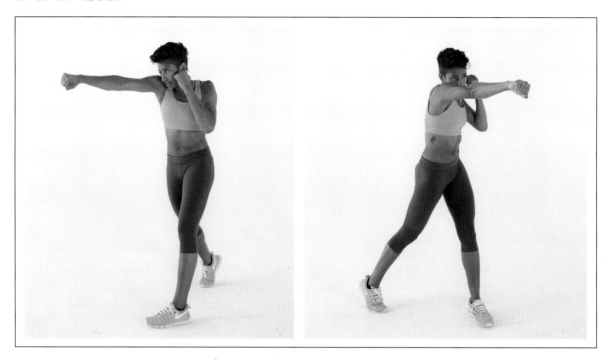

- In any punching combo, you will need to establish your stance.
- For a traditional boxing or kickboxing stance, your dominant side will become the rear side, with that leg standing behind and out at a 90-degree angle.
- If you are a righty, your right leg and arm will be back, and the left leg and arm will be forward.
- In fitness motions it is okay to switch leads.
- Bring your hands up, tuck your elbows in, and keep your knuckles at your cheeks, covering your jaw.
- Your rear leg will be on the ball of the foot.
- To throw a jab, you will extend your lead hand forward and turn your punch over (in a traditional jab).
- Your cross, or *straight right*, will come from the back hand.
- Reach over the rear arm and pivot on the rear foot as you turn your hip and reach the punch across your body, turning the punch over and aiming straight.
- Return the arm back and continue in a jab-cross combo.

JAB-CROSS-HOOK

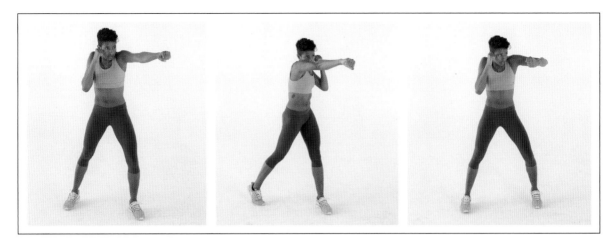

- You can perform a hook, or a looping punch, with either arm, rear or front.
- In a jab-cross combo, we will perform the motions by alternating arms—front, rear, and the hook with your front arm to maximize on your hips' torque.
- To add a hook to the punch combo previously discussed, complete a jab-cross, and then take your front hand and turn it at the elbow so that your shoulder and elbow line up, and your elbow lines up with the wrist.
- Pivot your lead foot and shift your hip to follow through with the hook.
- Return the arm back by the chin and continue to a jab-cross-hook combo.

JAB-CROSS-BODY HOOK

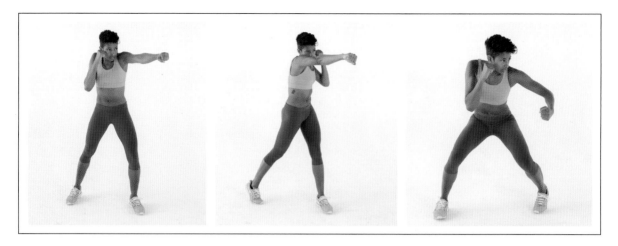

- In this jab-cross combo, we will perform the motions by alternating arms—front, rear, and the uppercut with your front arm to maximize on your hips' torque.

- To add a hook, complete a jab-cross, and then take your front hand and turn it at the elbow so that your shoulder and elbow line up, and your elbow lines up with the wrist.

- Dip down slightly as you shift your front foot and push up from the hip in an uppercut motion.

- Return the arm back by the chin and continue to a jab-cross-hook combo.

PUNCHING COMBOS TO PUSH-UP

- Perform any of the punching combos listed.

- Immediately after, jump or step back into a plank.

- Lower yourself down in any of the push-up variations listed earlier in this chapter.

- As you come back up to a plank, jump the feet back up to the arms and stand right up. For a modification, you can also step back up.

- Repeat.

LEOPARD TURN-OUT

- Your starting position will be on all fours, on your knees.
- Make sure that your elbows, shoulders, and wrists are in line.
- Maintain strong, tight abdominal muscles and a straight back.
- Lift your knees up, half an inch off the floor, if you can. The modified version is to stay on your knees.
- First try to hold it for 10 seconds to test your form.
- When you are ready, raise up your body slowly onto your toes and turn to one side, lifting one arm off the floor.
- Continue this left and right, stopping in the middle each time to make sure you maintain proper form.
- Abdominals should be tight (think of pulling your belly button into your spine). Pull your shoulders back.
- You should not feel any pressure in your arm or shoulder. If you do, it simply means you need to develop more core strength—so in the meantime, modify by sitting on the floor with each turn to reset the body.
- Yes! You are training your core and legs too, but the main burn will be in the shoulders, back, triceps, and biceps.

SURFER

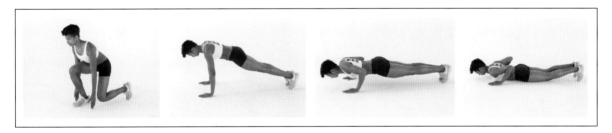

- Create a space in front of you and picture an imaginary surfboard. Drop down on the surfboard and lie down on it.
- With control, do a half push-up and push your upper body off of the floor.
- Continue by inserting your lower body and standing straight up on the surfboard.
- Repeat and drop back down on the board.
- Use your upper body, including the chest, back, arms, and abs.
- Make sure to envision yourself on the surfboard, and never rush past your form.

TURKISH GET-UP (TGU)

The **Turkish get-up** is a traditional kettlebell exercise. When you first start, I advise you to do the motion without a kettlebell (as pictured on the next page). The reason for this is simple: the TGU is done by holding the kettlebell overhead, which requires skill, knowledge of motion, and body awareness. Learn the six motions up and six down first, and then continue by adding kettlebell weight.

The Turkish get-up is a whole body exercise involving six steps to get from a faceup, lying-down position up to standing, and the same six steps back down. There are different types of TGUs that incorporate more or fewer steps (some of which we will illustrate in this book). What follows is the traditional TGU, beneficial for the core, legs, glutes, arms, and back as well as for mobility, stability, and strength.

Start with your back on the floor with your arm extended up off the ground, straight up (with or without a kettlebell in the hand of the extended arm; if you are not using a kettlebell, you should still act as if there is a kettlebell in your hand).

Form

- The arm never moves! Make sure it is overhead in a fixed position.
- Make sure you are staring at your kettlebell the entire time (never taking your eyes off of the bell until you are in a fully standing position).

Set-Up

- Your leg on the same side as the arm that is extended should be bent, while the other leg and arm are lying straight on the ground at about a 45-degree angle to your body.
- You must keep your shoulder blade packed back, and always keep your eyes on the kettlebell no matter what position you end up in (you can look forward only in the standing position).
- Your arm that is extended must also *always* stay up straight, perpendicular to the ground.

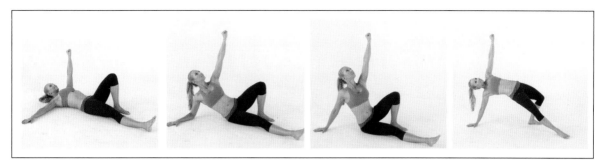

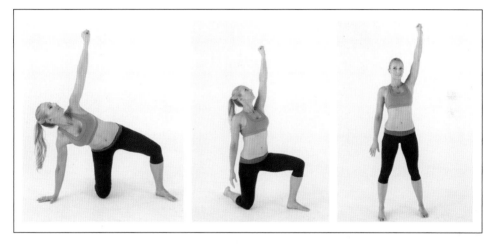

Start with the kettlebell in your left hand, left leg bent, in lying-down position.

1. Push yourself up to your right elbow.

2. Push yourself up to your right hand.

3. Lift your body up by pushing your hips up to the sky.

4. Swivel your right leg under your body and bend it so that you are now supported by your right knee, left foot, and right hand.

5. Come to a kneeling position by pushing off your right hand.

6. Come to a standing position with kettlebell secure overhead in your left hand.

Your TGU is not complete until you go down the same way you came up—illustrated here with a kettlebell.

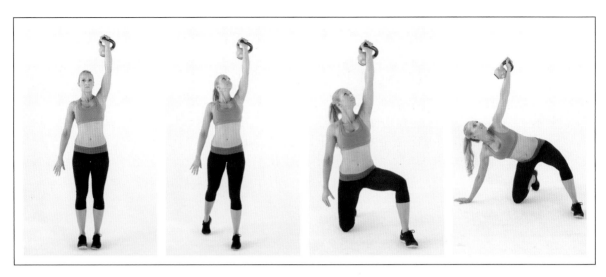

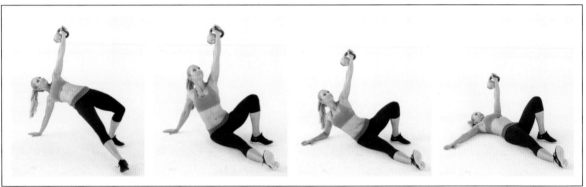

6 Steps to Get Down

1. Bring your right leg back to a kneeling position on the floor.

2. Put your right hand down by your side (**do not** position your hand too far back. This will make you sit on your right heel, which will make it harder for you to perform the next step where you have to move your right leg back out).

3. Swivel your right leg back out so that it is extended in front of you again (hips are still pushed up to the sky).

4. Bring your hips down so you are sitting on your butt.

5. Bring yourself down to your right elbow.

6. Lower yourself from your elbow so you are lying completely on the ground (your left arm should stay extended in the air if you are going to do multiple reps).

NOTE: To switch the kettlebell to the other side, do not cross it over your face. Bring the kettlebell down to your shoulder, place it on the ground next to you, and then, using both hands, drag the kettlebell on the floor around your head to the other side. Now you are ready to perform reps on the right side. Use your right hand to press the kettlebell up to the sky and bend your right leg while straightening out your left leg.

THE PERFECT UPPER BODY WORKOUT PLAN

Here are some options on how to put everything together for your workout to achieve a beautiful and strong upper body. They are in order from easiest to hardest.

For all workouts:
Start with 4–6 warm-up exercises from chapter 9.
End with 4–6 cool-down stretches from chapter 9.

Workout 1:

Complete 2 sets of any 8 exercises from this chapter.
Work with a challenging weight/pace (depending on the move) that will leave you sweating for 1 minute of work/30 seconds of rest between each set.

Workout 2:

Complete 3 sets of any 6 exercises from this chapter.
Work with a challenging weight at 8–15 reps per move.
You should feel challenged, and you should max out at the weight.

Workout 3:

Complete 4 sets of any 4 exercises from this chapter.
Work with a challenging weight/pace (depending on the move) that will leave you sweating for 1 minute of work/30 seconds of rest between each.

Workout 4:

Complete 2 sets of any 8 exercises from this chapter.
Work with a challenging weight at 8–15 reps per move.
You should feel challenged, and you should max out at the weight.

Workout 5:

Run a circuit of 8 exercises from this chapter.
Complete one full rotation of all 8 exercises: 1 minute work and 30 seconds rest.
Repeat the circuit one more time, but this time do 1 minute work and 15 seconds rest.

Workout 6:

Pick 6 exercises from this chapter and place them into the following module:

- Perform the first and second exercises you picked for 8 rounds of 20 seconds of work and 10 seconds of rest for a total of 4 minutes of work.
- Rest for 2 minutes (a more advanced routine cuts this down to 1 minute of rest).
- Perform the third and fourth exercises you picked for 8 rounds of 20 seconds of work and 10 seconds of rest for a total of 4 minutes of work.
- Rest for 2 minutes (a more advanced routine cuts this down to 1 minute of rest).
- Perform the fifth and sixth exercises you picked for 8 rounds of 20 seconds of work and 10 seconds of rest for a total of 4 minutes of work.
- Rest for 2 minutes (a more advanced routine cuts this down to 1 minute of rest).

Use the move listed or any of the move's variations:

Box A	Box B	Box C
Use any move from chapters 4, 7, or 8.	Use any move from chapter 6.	Use any move from chapter 5.

Pick 3 exercises from the boxes above; one exercise from Box A, one from Box B, and one from Box C.

Place them into the following module:

- Perform the first exercise you picked for 8 rounds of 20 seconds of work and 10 seconds of rest for a total of 4 minutes of work.
- Rest for 2 minutes (a more advanced routine cuts this down to 1 minute of rest).
- Perform the second exercise you picked for 8 rounds of 20 seconds of work and 10 seconds of rest for a total of 4 minutes of work.
- Rest for 2 minutes (a more advanced routine cuts this down to 1 minute of rest).
- Perform the third exercise you picked for 8 rounds of 20 seconds of work and 10 seconds of rest for a total of 4 minutes of work.
- Rest for 2 minutes (a more advanced routine cuts this down to 1 minute of rest).
- Stretch using 3–6 stretches from chapter 9.

CHAPTER 7

LIMITLESS LEGS

Cure Knee Pain and Sculpt Beautiful, Lean Legs

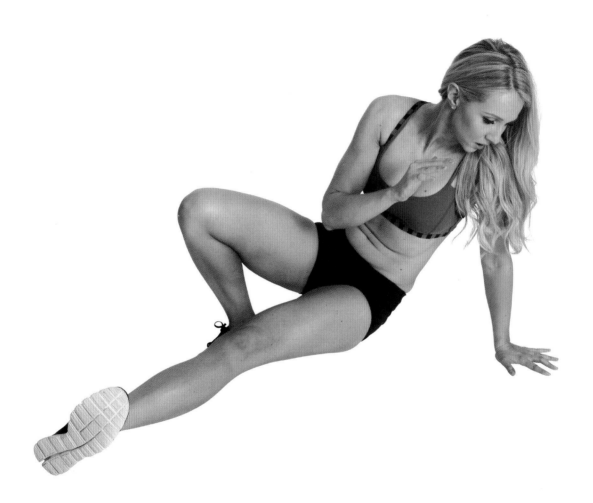

Legs are important; they help get you places. Plus, as women, we have the opportunity to show off our strong and sexy legs in dresses and shorts. It is for these reasons that you should never overlook your leg exercises. Plus, leg exercise burns more calories because you are working large muscles! Engaging the hamstrings, quadriceps, and calves takes a lot of energy, and a huge amount of exertion yields a high calorie burn. Strengthening the legs correctly with both quad- and hip-dominant motions will balance your body and fortify it, preventing overuse injuries and making you stronger in your sport and in your life. Smart leg workouts and exercises also strengthen the ligaments and tendons within your legs, helping make your knees and ankles more stable and less susceptible to injury or overuse.

BONUS! Make sure you hit all of the vital movement patterns for balanced, healthy legs. When your workout includes exercise like the kettlebell swing, the squat, lunges, and hip thrusters, you are also working countless other muscles in your body, including your core.

Remember that running is a sport, and not outright exercise. To get the right length tension relationships in the body and avoid injury and overuse, make sure you supplement your recreational activities with strength and conditioning exercises. Therefore, as much as you might think you are sculpting your legs when you run, you must lift weights and use resistance training to truly define your body, legs included!

LEG ANATOMY

FRONT OF THE LEG

Quadriceps: these are the main large muscles in the front of your thigh.

Hip adductors: these include a variety of muscles that shape the inner thigh. These muscles help move the hip and knee joints as well as balance the pelvis.

CALVES

Gastrocnemius: helps you bend the knee and is also responsible for that beautiful shape of the calf.

Soleus: this part of the calf is capable of extending a force on the ankle, helping us push off the ground when we walk or run, or stand on our toes.

BACK OF THE LEG

Hamstrings: your hamstrings are actually composed of three muscles. The hamstrings bend the knee and help your glutes extend the hip (that is why so many exercises work the hamstrings and the glutes simultaneously). They also help rotate the thigh inward and outward.

YOUR EXERCISES!

SINGLE-ARM KETTLEBELL SWING

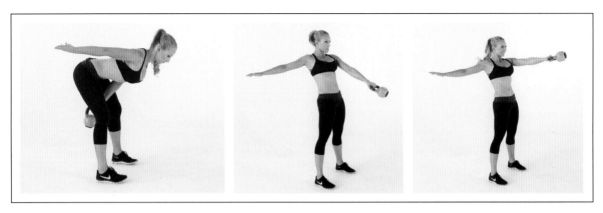

As we've seen from the previous chapters, the kettlebell swing is an incredible posterior chain exercise that also does wonders for the core and for calorie burn. However, a big part of the posterior chain is the legs, so it's important to make sure you know that you can place your kettlebell swing in your leg workouts.

We will get to the traditional two-handed swing in the glutes chapter (8), but first we'll introduce the single-arm swing in this Limitless Legs chapter.

- The fundamental part of this motion is the traditional kettlebell swing, using one arm instead of two.

- The only difference between the traditional kettlebell swing and the single-arm kettlebell swing is that when your arm goes back and behind the knees to swing, you must make sure that your thumb is facing back, not up in front of you. This secures a good and safe arm position.

- Pick up the kettlebell by the handle and sit back, bending first at the hips, then at the knees in a hinge.

- As you hinge and swing the kettlebell back and behind the knees, thrust your hips forward and raise your torso back to the standing position, then continue without stopping back down into your hinge again.

- Create a nonstop, fluid motion of the swing; the kettlebell will go behind the knees and back up to shoulder level.

- Do not raise the kettlebell with your arms. The kettlebell should feel weightless in your arms throughout the entire motion.

- Squeeze your glutes as you push your hips forward, making sure your butt muscles are engaged and working.
- Do not backward bend at the top of the motion.
- At the top of the swing, remember to keep your arms straight, thrust your hips forward, straighten your knees, and swing the kettlebell no higher than chest level as you rise to standing position and engage the glutes (squeeze the butt muscles together).

SQUAT

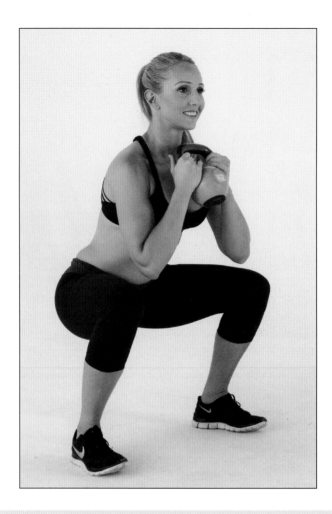

This is also traditionally called the kettlebell goblet squat, where the kettlebell is held in goblet position.

- Hold the kettlebell in mid-racked position.
- As you inhale, pull yourself down with tension into a full squat.
- Keep as flat as possible, torso erect, ears over shoulders, and knee caps tracked over toes.
- The weight should be on the heels, not the front of the foot.
- The angle of the feet varies from individual to individual.
- Push the knees with the elbows, if needed, to keep them tracked properly.
- On the exhale, without leaning forward, stand erect.

Change your kettlebell grips for some diversity of movement with one of these options (see chapter 2 for a review of kettlebell grips):

- Hold the kettlebell in a goblet position (with the base facing up, holding the bell between your palms).

- Hold your kettlebell with one arm in a racked position.

- For a super challenge and **core bonus**, hold your single kettlebell with the bottoms-up grip (holding the handle by the horns, with the base facing up).

TRY THIS KETTLEBELL BONUS TRANSITION:

- Swing the kettlebell from a good hinge up and catch on the palm of the hand with the elbow tight to the ribs.

- Catch and position the kettlebell in a goblet position.

OVERHEAD SQUAT

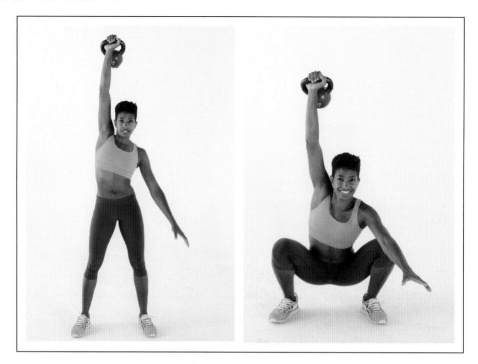

Please note that this is an advanced motion. Beginners should start out without a kettlebell, using only the arms. Once this feels comfortable and your form is correct, you can try it with a kettlebell. More advanced is the double kettlebell overhead squat, executed the same way, but with two kettlebells (one in each hand).

- For beginners, start out doing this move using no kettlebell (just your arms).
- With a kettlebell, make sure to have a grip on the handle, with the belly of the bell resting on your forearm in a racked position.
- Press the racked kettlebell overhead, with your arm straight.
- Make sure your abdominals are tight and your shoulders are sitting back.
- Set your feet shoulders' width apart in a starting squat position.
- Do not at any point allow the arm, or the kettlebell, to move forward as you lower your body down into a squat.
- Keep your lower back naturally arched and your shoulders packed and pulled back.
- Your arm should stay perpendicular to the floor for the entire lift.
- Drive through your heels on the way back up, never moving the arm.

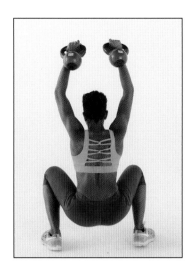

ADVANCED: More advanced is the double kettlebell overhead squat, executed the same exact way, but with two kettlebells.

SQUAT TO SNAP KICK

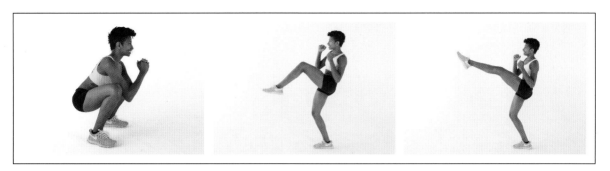

- You can choose to do the motion without a kettlebell, or holding a kettle-bell in a mid-racked position.

- Perform the traditional squat, with or without a kettlebell.

- Every time you return back to standing position, bring one leg up and bend it at the knee as you snap up the leg in one swift motion.

- Return back to standing on both legs in a squat-ready stance and squat back down.

- Alternate legs.

- Note that if you are holding a kettlebell, keep it chest level, mid-racked, or (for doubles) racked the entire time.

JUMP SQUAT

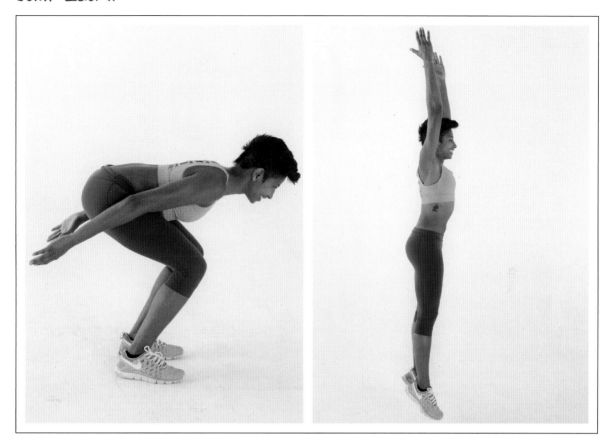

- As you execute this motion, go back in a hinge rather than a traditional squat.
- In a squat thruster like the one involved in a jump squat, you must hinge so that you can use your glutes to push off.
- Sit back and bring your hips back. Then bend the knees.
- Push off of the heels and jump up in a vertical jump.
- Land lightly and do not pound at the knees or joints.

THRUSTER

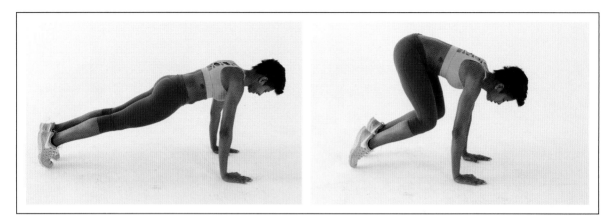

- Jump back from standing into a plank.
- Jump back up to standing.
- Keep your core tight and maintain proper form in your plank.
- To make the motion more difficult, jump both feet up to one side of your arms.
- You can also add a variation of push-ups to the mix, as well as a jump squat (making it a burpee).

SUMO SQUAT

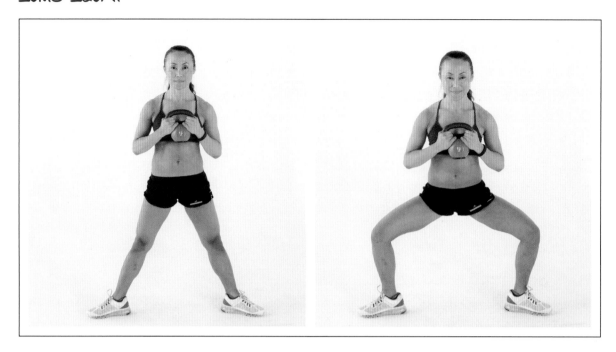

- Hold a kettlebell in a mid-racked position.
- Set your feet wider than you would in a squat, with each toe about a foot out from under the shoulder.
- You feet should be at a 45-degree external rotation.
- Keep your back straight and your shoulder blades pulled back.
- Perform the same exact movement as a squat.

DOUBLE KB SUMO SQUAT

- Complete the same exact motion, except you will have two kettlebells racked.

Change your kettlebell grips for some diversity of movement with one of these options:

- Hold the kettlebell in a goblet position.
- Hold your kettlebell with one arm in a racked position.
- For a super challenge and **core bonus**, hold your single kettlebell with the bottoms-up grip (holding the handle by the horns, with the base facing up).

ADD THIS TO YOUR SQUATS AND SUMO SQUATS:

Core Killer Grip: Another super advanced option is to have two kettlebells in bottoms-up position, held steady and close to the body as the entire motion is performed.

KILLER COMBO

- Hold the kettlebell mid-racked position.
- As you inhale, pull yourself down with tension into a full squat.
- Keep your back as flat as possible, torso erect, ears over shoulders, and knee caps tracked over toes.
- The weight should be on the heels, not the front of the foot; you should be able to wiggle your toes at any point.
- On the exhale, without leaning forward, push right back up and onto your toes.
- At the same time as you push up, press the kettlebell overhead.
- Then lower back down into a squat, and this time as you push back up, turn to the left and pivot your right foot as you push the kettlebell overhead.
- Continue back down and then come back up, this time turning to the other side.
- Once all three motions are complete, you have successfully performed one rep.

KARATE SUMO SQUAT HOLD

You can execute this move with or without a kettlebell.

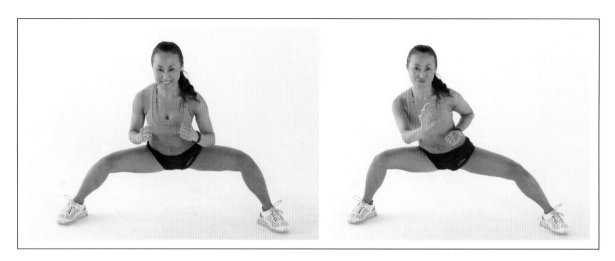

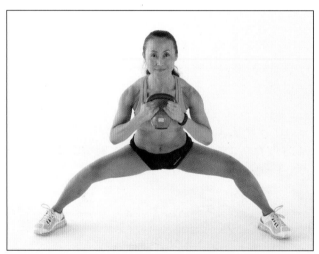

- Complete the sumo squat.
- On your next rep, stay in the bottom position and hold.
- You should aim to press inward with your feet, keeping your heels pressed firmly into the ground.
- Aim to get deeper and deeper and deeper into the squat, all while keeping your core tight.
- Your goal is a 1-minute hold.
- While you hold, you can move your upper body an inch or two to the left and right.

SUMO JACK

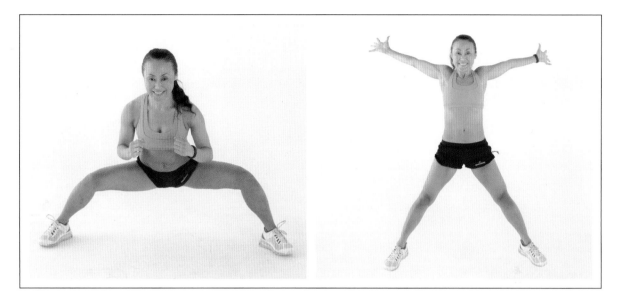

- Hold the sumo squat for a count of 10 seconds.
- Explode from your heels to a jumping jack in which you push high off of the ground in a full jump.

SUMO SQUAT TO CRESCENT KICK

- Between each sumo squat, complete a crescent kick as you come up to starting position.
- Keep your back strong and straight and your core tight.

SPLIT SUMO

- Complete a sumo squat, but as you do, reach one arm out to touch the floor.
- The other arm should be reaching up, extended overhead, strong and straight.

SPEED SKATER

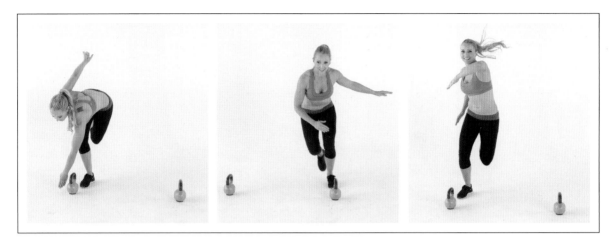

- Using single-leg dead lift form, balance on one foot as you reach over with the opposite hand and touch the floor.
- Jump (pushing off of your stationary leg) to the other side, landing on the other foot.
- Reach over with the opposite hand.
- Repeat nonstop with a strong and straight back, jumping from one side to the other.
- Maintain your form and your balance.

JINGA LUNGES

- This is similar to a speed skater, just with a deep lunge.
- Start on one side and take a deep rear lunge back.
- Push off of the front leg and take a hop to the other leg as you jump to the side.
- You are jumping and at the same time switching the feet of your lunge.
- Repeat nonstop with a strong and straight back, jumping from one side to the other.
- Maintain your form and your balance.

LATERAL HOPS

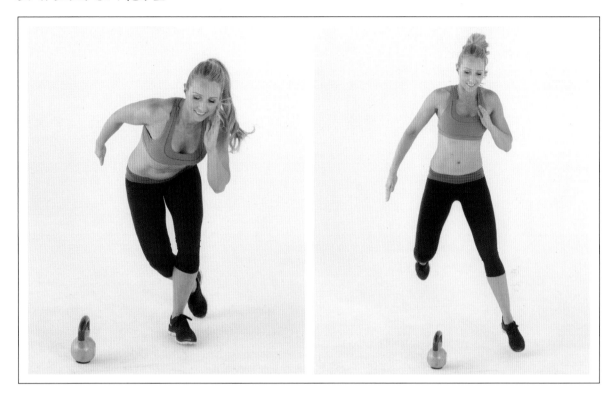

- Place one kettlebell on the floor.
- Hop from one side to the other nonstop, with no tension on the knees.
- Use your arms to help you push off and generate power.
- Make sure to land lightly on the feet.

FOOT FIRE SPRAWL

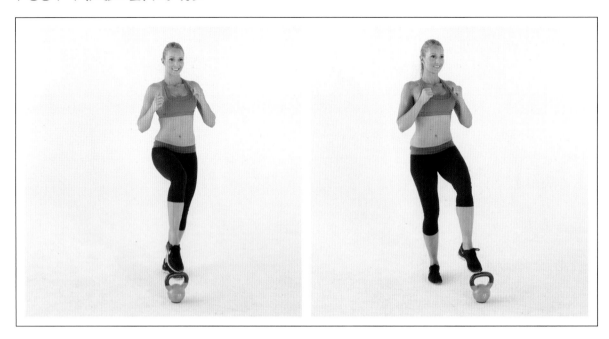

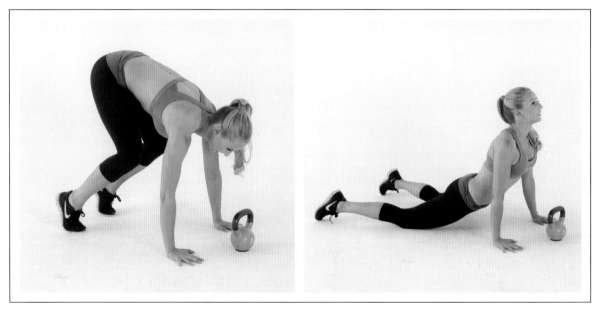

- Place a kettlebell in front of you.
- With no pressure on the knees, alternate light hops.
- As you lift the foot, touch it to the handle of the kettlebell without letting it fall.
- Execute 4 touches and continue down to the sprawl (detailed in full in chapter 8).

KNEE SKIP-UPS

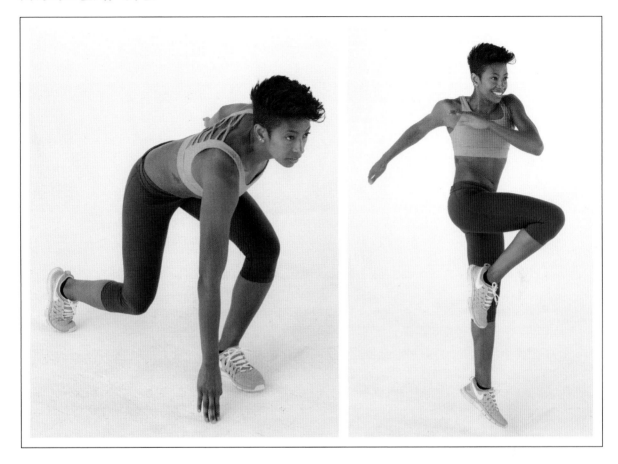

These are a little more ballistic than the knees we learned in the abs chapter; because there is a lot of drive through the legs, this move works for a legs routine.

- Stand in your kickboxing stance.
- Now step back into a deeper stance, almost like a rear lunge, and touch the floor with one arm.
- Take your rear leg and drive it up, bending it at the knee so that you are driving, pushing, and single-leg jumping.
- Push the crown of your knee forward and up.
- As you step back, make sure that you step back into your kickboxing stance.
- Always knee with the rear leg starting from your kickboxing stance.
- This should feel like you are skipping out of a deep lunge up into the air.
- Only when you get comfortable, add a light hop/skip to the knee.

KB WARRIOR

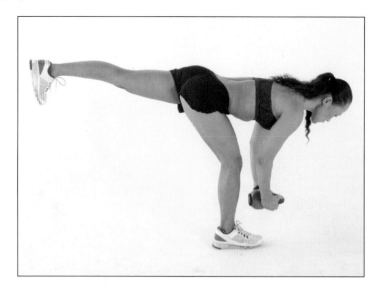

- Pick up the kettlebell with two hands and stand erect, kettlebell at mid-racked position.
- Fold the waist and sit back as the hips travel backward.
- Maintain a flat back, and on the inhale lower the kettlebell close to the ground.
- At the same time, begin kicking the other leg back behind you in a straight line with your back.
- From the side, your body should look like a T, with the arms and kettlebell hanging down in front of you.
- The working leg can bend slightly as you fold forward, with no hyperextension.

NON-KB WARRIOR

- You can also perform the warrior without a kettlebell.
- This time, instead of bringing the arms down to the floor, stretch them out and in front of you (in a straight line with the hips, in even more of a T shape than with the kettlebell).

LUNGE

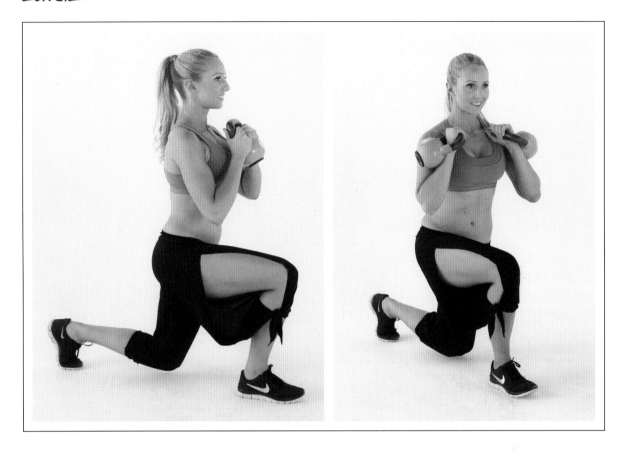

Lunges include the rear (or split-squat lunge), lateral lunge, walking lunge, crescent lunge, and alternating lunge.

- Hold a kettlebell chest level in a mid-racked position.
- Other hold options are: goblet, bottoms-up, racked (single kettlebell with one arm), and double-racked (double kettlebells).
- Stand in a straight line, with abdominals tight, a strong core, and a straight back.
- Step forward on the ball of your back foot and sink into the heel of the stepping foot.
- Keeping your torso as upright as possible, slowly lower your body as far as you can.
- Your rear knee should nearly touch the floor, or it can touch the floor if needed.
- Pause, then push yourself back up, driving through the heel of the stepping leg to the starting position as quickly as you can.

You can change it up by holding the kettlebell with these grips:

- Goblet
- Mid-racked (as described)
- Double kettlebells mid-racked
- Single-arm racked
- Hanging to one side (the side and arm opposite the lunge; back must stay straight)
- Two kettlebells, one hanging to each side
- Bottoms-up (advanced)

WALKING LUNGE

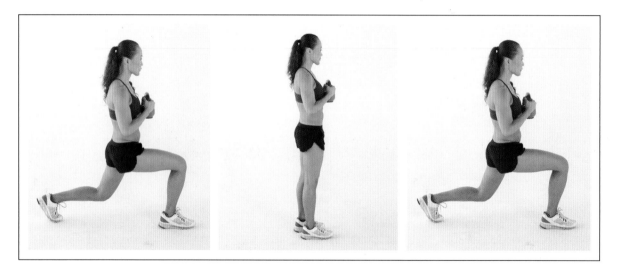

- You should perform the same exact motion as illustrated in the lunge, except when it comes time to step back to starting position; instead, you will simply step through and continue to lunge forward.
- In walking lunges it is traditional to have one or two kettlebells hanging at your sides; however, any of the other holds are great options.

REVERSE LUNGE

- Hold the kettlebell in the same position as in the goblet squat.
- Step back with the right foot.
- Touch the right knee gently to the ground. The thigh should be parallel to the ground.
- The front knee should track over the toes, and the torso should be vertical.
- Return to the standing position on the exhale.
- Press though the heel and bring the back leg up and in line.

WARRIOR LUNGE

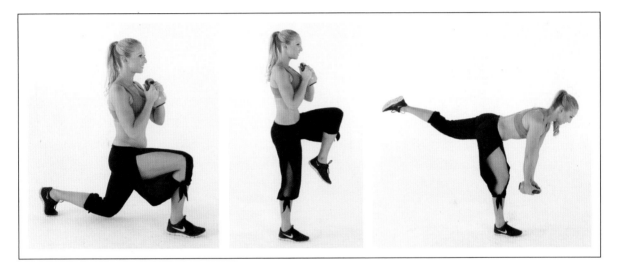

- Perform the reverse lunge with the kettlebell mid-racked.
- Pushing off of the leg, continue on to the front leg and go right into a KB warrior.
- Come back up from the warrior to starting position and continue on to the next lunge-warrior combo.

PISTON SQUAT

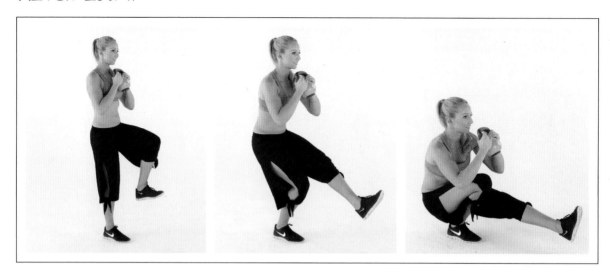

ADVANCED: You should note that the piston squat, with or without the kettlebell, is a very advanced motion and should not be performed unless you have strong and balanced glutes and legs, including no knee pain or instability. The motion is shown in this book specifically because it is traditional to kettlebells. However a lunge, split squat, or squat is just as beneficial.

- To perform the move without a kettlebell, stand holding your arms straight out in front of your body at shoulder level, parallel to the floor.
- If you are ready to move on to trying it with a kettlebell, hold the kettlebell in a mid-racked position.
- Raise your right leg off the floor and hold it there.
- Sit back in a single-leg squat, with the other leg extended directly in front of you.
- Sit back and lower your body as far as you can.
- As you lower your body, raise your right leg so that it doesn't touch the floor—this takes balance, strength, and mobility.
- Do not force it.
- Keep your torso as upright as possible, with your shoulders pulled back.
- You must push through your heel on the way up, making sure your heel is never off of the ground.

- Drive up through your glute muscles.
- Pause, then push your body back to the starting position.

Modified piston squat can include the following options:
- Use a wall and place one hand on it for balance and support.
- Begin from the ground, in a single-leg dead lift, and use your arm to help you up.

LATERAL LUNGE

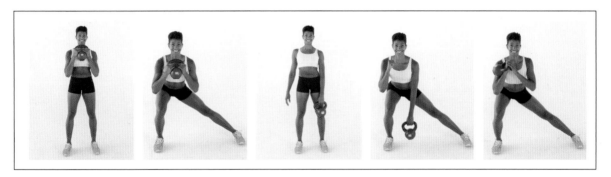

- Hold a kettlebell in mid-racked position (photos 1 and 2), hanging (photos 3 and 4), or just racked (photo 5).
- Tighten your core and make sure that your back is straight and strong.
- Stand tall with your feet hips' width apart.
- Lift your right foot and take a big step to your right as you push your hips backward; lower your body by dropping your hips and bending your left knee.
- Make sure your right hip, knee, and foot are lined up.
- Push yourself back up to the starting position.
- You can stay on one side and alternate.
- If you have the kettlebell mid-racked or racked, the kettlebell will remain fixed and never move away from your torso.
- Your heel should always be rooted into the ground, never coming up and off of the floor.
- Push off of your heel as you come up and out of the lateral lunge.
- You can alternate sides or stay on one side.

LATERAL LUNGE AND LIFT

- As you perform the lunge on one side, keep the kettlebell at mid-racked position.
- When you come back to starting position, lift the kettlebell up overhead in a double-arm press.
- Then lower the kettlebell as you step over to the other side.
- Continue in a lunge-lift-lunge-lift rhythm, but without compromising speed for form.

DOUBLE KB LATERAL LUNGE

- Hold two kettlebells in a racked position, firm and tight to the body.
- Perform the same exact motion as the lateral lunge.
- Never move the bells.

CRESCENT SQUAT

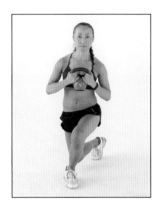

- Hold a kettlebell mid-racked.
- Instead of stepping directly behind you when you lunge, cross your foot behind and over to the side as if you were doing a curtsy.
- Step back to center and continue on one side or alternating.
- Other options include holding the kettlebell in a goblet, holding it single racked, or using two double-racked kettlebells.

CRESCENT SQUAT TO CRESCENT KICK

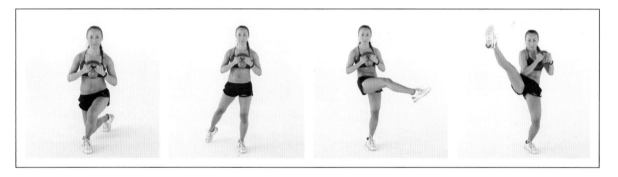

- Perform the same exact motion as described in the crescent squat.
- At the end (top) of the motion, stop and bring the leg that was behind you out to the side.
- Touch the floor for a second and continue to perform a crescent kick.
- In a crescent kick, you will be kicking in a circle away from the body.
- Reset back to starting position and start over.
- The kettlebell should never move from being mid-racked in front of your chest.

45-DEGREE REAR LUNGE

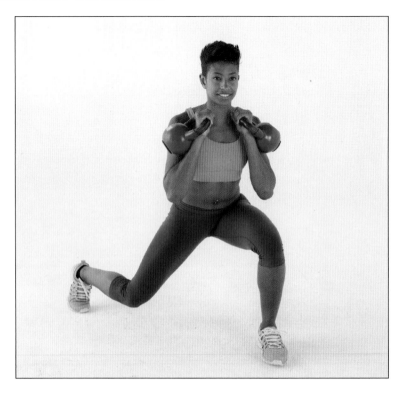

- Hold a kettlebell mid-racked.
- Instead of stepping straight forward, lunge back diagonally at a 45-degree angle outward.
- Other options include holding the kettlebell in a goblet, holding it single racked, or using two double-racked kettlebells (as shown here).

3-WAY LUNGE

- Step back into a rear lunge.
- Then step to a crescent lunge out of the rear lunge.
- Then continue to the 45-degree lunge from the crescent.

KB REAR LUNGE TO PUSH KICK

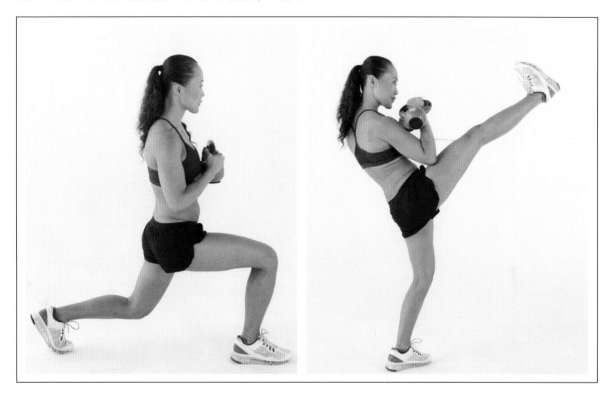

- Complete a rear lunge with the kettlebell mid-racked.
- As you come up, stop at the top of the lunge and bring the rear leg through and up into a push kick.
- The kettlebell should never move from its position.
- For a more challenging version, go directly from the rear lunge to the kick, without the stop in the middle.
- For a bonus challenge, raise the kettlebell overhead on the way up with your kick.
- Even more challenging would be to bring the kettlebell overhead as you come into the lunge.

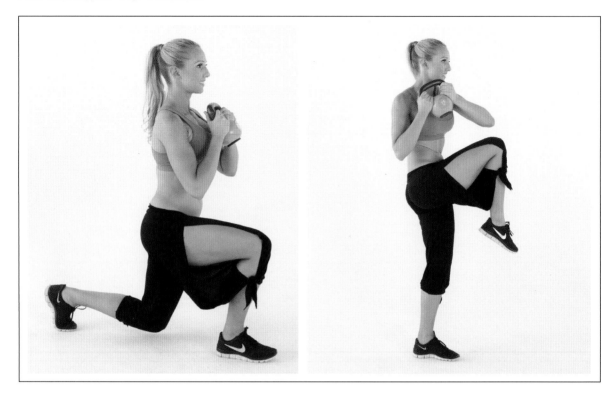

- Complete a rear lunge with the kettlebell mid-racked.
- As you come up, stop at the top of the lunge, bringing the rear leg through and up, leading with your knee.
- As you bring the knee up, move your shoulders toward the kneeing leg in a slight twist (originating from your shoulders).
- The kettlebell should never move from its position without your shoulders.
- For a more challenging version, go directly from the rear lunge to the knee, without the stop in the middle.
- Even more challenging would be to bring the kettlebell overhead as you come back into a lunge and then go into the knee.

LUNGE AND PRESS

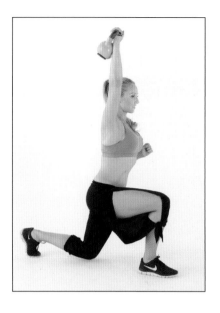

- Complete a rear lunge with the kettlebell racked to one side, with one arm.
- As you lunge back, simultaneously raise the arm with the kettlebell into a press.
- As you come back up out of the lunge, bring the arm back to racked position.

KB OVERHEAD REAR LUNGE

- Hold a kettlebell in the mid-racked position.
- Keep your core tight and your back strong and straight.
- As you go into a rear lunge, raise the kettlebell overhead and straighten your arms.
- Complete the lunge.
- Make sure to drive through your heel on the way up, and as you come up, lower the kettlebell back to chest level in mid-racked position.
- Do not allow the kettlebell to move as you bring it overhead. Keep it fixed and stable.
- Keep your torso upright for the entire movement.

BONUS! You can also perform the motion with double kettlebells.

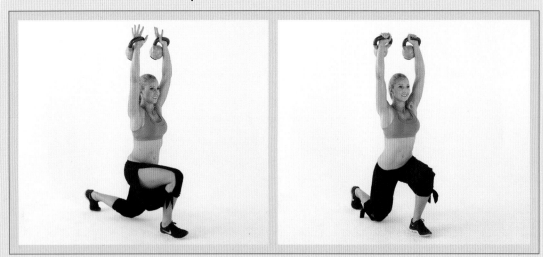

- Press both kettlebells up at the same time as you perform the lunge back.
- Another option would be to alternate the overhead press with single or double kettlebells, keeping one kettlebell racked while the other comes up on the rear lunge.

CAT SQUAT

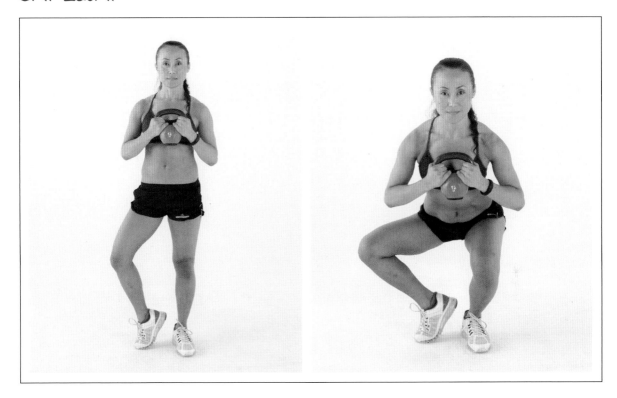

- Stand straight up; the kettlebell can be racked or mid-racked, tight to the body.
- Bring your feet together as you face forward.
- Take one foot and rotate it out so it is 90 degrees out from the other foot.
- Make sure that both of your heels are still touching each other.
- From there, take the foot that is rotated out and come up on your toe as high as possible.
- Now keep the foot in this position and begin to squat down into that leg, flexing the calf and really making sure that all of the weight of the squatting leg is in your toe.
- You should feel your inner thigh the entire time.
- It should look like a half plié.

KB CALF RAISE

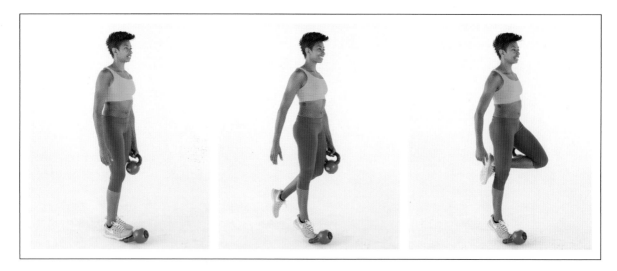

- You will need two kettlebells, one as a prop and the other as a weight.
- Place the larger kettlebell (or one of the kettlebells, if you don't have more than one weight of kettlebells) on the ground in front of you.
- Hold a kettlebell by the handle at your left side, with your palm facing inward and your thumb forward.
- Place your right toe on the handle of the bell on the ground. Your left heel should be off of the bell, on the ground at the start.
- Cross your left foot behind your right ankle or lift it slightly so that you are balancing on a single foot.
- If needed, place one hand on something stable like a wall, while the other hand holds the kettlebell.
- Lift your heel as high as you can, flexing your calf.
- Pause, then lower and repeat in a controlled lift each time.
- Switch sides.

SPLIT JUMPS

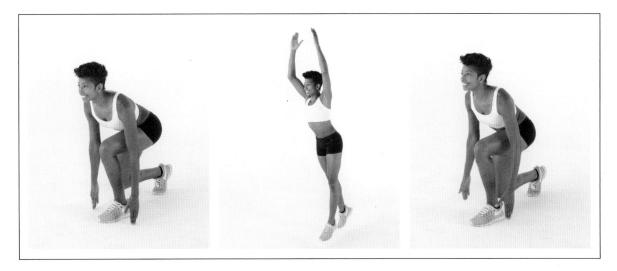

- Make sure that you have good knees and no injuries when you perform this motion.
- Establish a lead leg and step the other leg behind you in a comfortable, wide side stance.
- Squat down using your glutes, and legs.
- Push off of the ground and jump up, switching the legs in the air and landing with the opposite leg forward (basically switching your stance).
- To perform a modified version of this motion, step and switch your stance instead of jumping.

Add a Kick to your Split Jump

- It's always nice to add a bonus motion to something as simple as the split squat.
- Try adding the push or snap kicks, kicking with the rear leg right before you push off to switch.
- Adding a knee, or several knees, can also add a bonus muscle activator and give the motion some individuality.
- Knee once, twice, or three times with the rear leg, bringing the leg across the body and up.
- After you bring the kneeing leg back to your split-squat stance, complete one or three split squats.

LEOPARD KICK-OUT

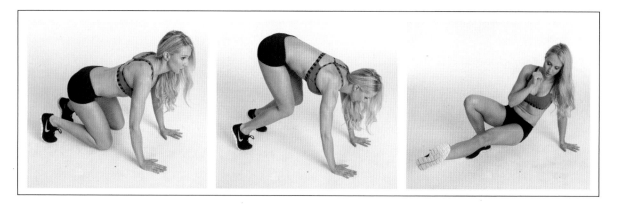

- Starting position is on all fours, on your knees, as pictured. Your elbows, shoulders, and wrists should be in line.

- Maintain strong, tight abdominal muscles and a straight back; lift your knees up, half an inch off the floor.

- Make sure you are still at 90-degree angles, not lifting your butt higher than the rest of your body.

- This is a tough position, so first, first try to hold it for 10 seconds to test your form.

- When you are ready, raise up your body slowly onto your toes and turn to one side, lifting one arm off the floor (as shown above). Continue this left and right, stopping in the middle each time to make sure you maintain proper form.

- Your abdominals should be tight (think of pulling your belly button into your spine) and your shoulders should be pulled back.

- You should feel no pressure in your arm or shoulder. If you do, it simply means we need to develop more core strength—so in the meantime modify by sitting on the floor with each turn to reset the body.

- After completing several leopard turns, continue to the leopard kick-out. Please note that if you cannot maintain good form on the first three motions, do not advance to the kick-out (instead work only with the first two motions illustrated in the first two photos above).

- In the leopard kick-out, you will simply kick your leg out (as shown in the third photo) as you turn your body.

- Continue this motion for 1 minute, or until you can no longer maintain proper form to execute the motion. Or continue this motion for the prescribed number of reps/sets or time intervals your KB workout calls for!

KB CHOP

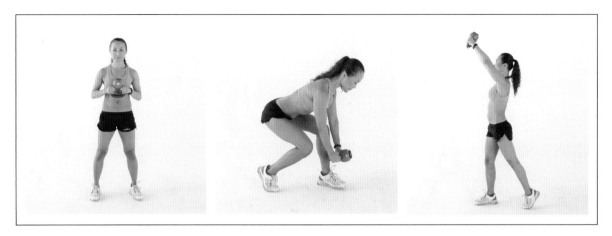

While this motion hits the abs and arms, the primary focus you will feel will be in your glutes, hamstrings, and legs.

- Mid-rack a kettlebell and hold it with both hands at chest level in starting position.
- Set your feet shoulders' width apart.
- Rotate your torso to your right and pivot your feet to the right as well.
- Your arms should now be straight and facing the floor.
- Keep your core muscles tight and engaged.
- Your right foot should have a hinge and a mild bend to it, not in a full extension and not in a squat, but a hinge (similar to a single-leg dead lift).
- Bring the kettlebell down and to the outside of your left knee by rotating to the left and bending at your hips.
- Don't round your lower back; keep it strong and straight.
- Reverse the movement to return to the start position; then rotate and pivot the feet to the opposite side and raise the kettlebell overhead with both hands.
- Continue the motion left to right and then right to left on the other side.

THE PERFECT LEG WORKOUT PLAN

Here are some options on how to put everything together for your workout to achieve beautiful and strong legs. They are in order from easiest to hardest.

For all workouts:
Start with 4–6 warm-up exercises from chapter 9.
End with 4–6 cool-down stretches from chapter 9.

Workout 1:

Complete 2 sets of any 8 exercises from this chapter.
Work with a challenging weight/pace (depending on the move) that will leave you sweating for 1 minute of work/30 seconds of rest between each set.

Workout 2:

Complete 3 sets of any 6 exercises from this chapter.
Work with a challenging weight at 8–15 reps per move.
You should feel challenged, and you should max out at the weight.

Workout 3:

Complete 4 sets of any 4 exercises from this chapter.
Work with a challenging weight/pace (depending on the move) that will leave you sweating for 1 minute of work/30 seconds of rest between each.

Workout 4:

Complete 2 sets of any 8 exercises from this chapter.
Work with a challenging weight at 8–15 reps per move.
You should feel challenged, and you should max out at the weight.

Workout 5:

Run a circuit of 8 exercises from this chapter.
Complete one full rotation of all 8 exercises: 1 minute work and 30 seconds rest.
Repeat the circuit one more time, but this time do 1 minute work and 15 seconds rest.

Workout 6:

Pick 6 exercises from this chapter and place them into the following module:

- Perform the first and second exercises you picked for 8 rounds of 20 seconds of work and 10 seconds of rest for a total of 4 minutes of work.
- Rest for 2 minutes (a more advanced routine cuts this down to 1 minute of rest).
- Perform the third and fourth exercises you picked for 8 rounds of 20 seconds of work and 10 seconds of rest for a total of 4 minutes of work.
- Rest for 2 minutes (a more advanced routine cuts this down to 1 minute of rest).
- Perform the fifth and sixth exercises you picked for 8 rounds of 20 seconds of work and 10 seconds of rest for a total of 4 minutes of work.
- Rest for 2 minutes (a more advanced routine cuts this down to 1 minute of rest).

Use the move listed or any of the move's variations:

Box A	Box B	Box C
Use any move from chapters 4, 7, or 8.	Use any move from chapter 6.	Use any move from chapter 5.

Pick 3 exercises from the boxes above; one exercise from Box A, one from Box B, and one from Box C.

Place them into the following module:
- Perform the first exercise you picked for 8 rounds of 20 seconds of work and 10 seconds of rest for a total of 4 minutes of work.
- Rest for 2 minutes (a more advanced routine cuts this down to 1 minute of rest).
- Perform the second exercise you picked for 8 rounds of 20 seconds of work and 10 seconds of rest for a total of 4 minutes of work.
- Rest for 2 minutes (a more advanced routine cuts this down to 1 minute of rest).
- Perform the third exercise you picked for 8 rounds of 20 seconds of work and 10 seconds of rest for a total of 4 minutes of work.
- Rest for 2 minutes (a more advanced routine cuts this down to 1 minute of rest).
- Stretch using 3–6 stretches from chapter 9.

CHAPTER 8

MAXIMIZE YOUR GLUTES

Building a Better Butt for Sports, Life, and Your Jeans

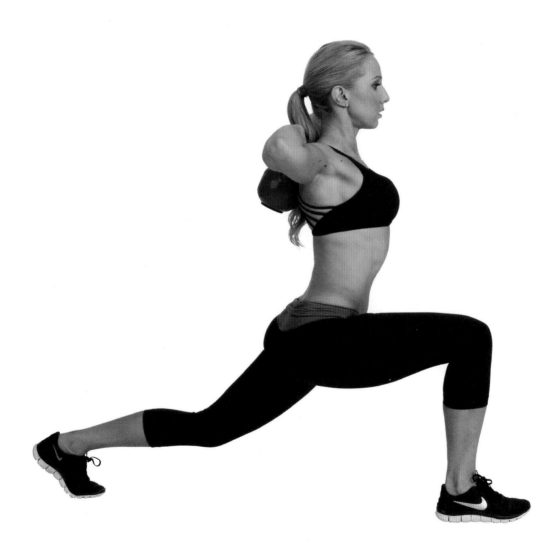

If one were to name a powerhouse of muscles in the body, one could strongly argue that your glutes are those muscles! **So, yes, it's actually okay that you spend so much time thinking about lifting, sculpting, and training your way to a better bottom.**

However, the sad fact is that many of us have tried to train our buttocks, and have seen little to no real results. But before you blame genetics, blame the modern lifestyle! And then—fix it. The truth is that as much as we care about this area of the body, it is commonly overlooked in many of our conditioning routines! Why? It's because after we spend the bulk of our day sitting at work, during our commute, and after work during our relaxation time, the glutes cease to "fire" or activate during basic motions they were designed to do like hinge, run, squat, and lunge. Therefore, when we go to the gym and think we are working our glutes, many of us barely accomplish a simple activation of that area of the body; our muscles have long forgotten how to contract during hip motion. Instead, all of the stress is placed into our knees, and we often leave our lower body workouts or cardio sessions feeling weaker and in pain (ankles, knees, and back) instead of energized and strong.

The much-needed hip-dominant gluteal muscle (buttocks) exercises are commonly left out of strength programs. Many people automatically assume they are working their gluteal muscles during running and squatting—but too often they are not activating those muscles! As an example, traditionally when we run, the glutes hold our pelvis, extend our hip, propel us forward, and keep our legs, pelvis, and torso aligned. But when our glutes are not activated, our entire kinetic chain gets disrupted, we use the wrong muscles to push ourselves forward in running, and we develop overuse injuries and pain. Studies have linked glute weakness to ankle, knee, back, and even neck injuries.

It is very important to work the glute muscle with hinge motions, as we will demonstrate in this chapter. It is also very important to distinguish your quad and your hip-dominant movement patterns and include both in your training. The kettlebell swing, the dead lift, good mornings, and hip thrusters are all wonderful hinge motions that will help activate your glutes.

> **BONUS!** Get a greater calorie burn when activating your glutes! Since the glutes are your biggest muscle group, they're also one of your top calorie burners. What's more, most glute exercises require you to activate your abdominal and lower back muscles in order to keep your body stable, so you get a bonus ab and back workout too!

YOUR BUTTOCKS: GLUTEAL ANATOMY

Gluteus maximus: this is the guy that creates that wonderful circular shape we all want and work so hard for. You work this muscle anytime you raise your thigh out to the side, rotate your leg, or thrust forward. This muscle also helps you lift up, from being in a chair to getting out of a squat.

Gluteus medius and **gluteus minimus:** these guys help stabilize the pelvis and help the gluteus maximus rotate your thigh out to the side.

> It is difficult not to include your hamstrings with the glutes, as they so commonly work together and are also activated together during common exercises. This is the reason we have included the hamstrings in this chapter, and many exercises will be working the glutes and hamstrings simultaneously.

Hamstrings: your hamstrings are actually composed of three muscles, including the **semitendinosus**, the **semimembranosus**, and the **biceps femoris**. The hamstrings bend the knee and help your glutes extend the hip (that is why so many exercises work both the hamstrings and glutes simultaneously). They also help rotate the thigh inward and outward.

YOUR EXERCISES!
ALL SWING FORM

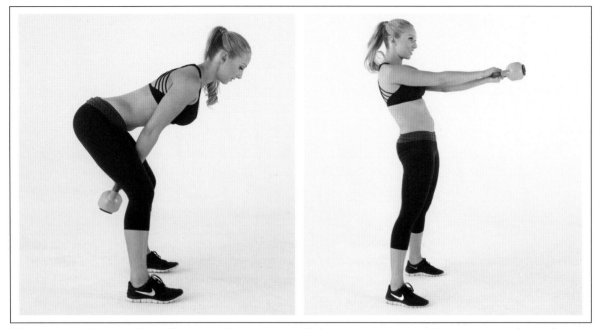

Note that the kettlebell swing is an incredible posterior chain exercise that also does wonders for the core and for calorie burn.

Let's review the traditional two-handed swing first seen in chapter 4—it is fundamental to every swing listed in this chapter.

1. With both hands, pick up the kettlebell by the handle and sit back in a hinge, bending first and more deeply at the hips, then at the knees.

2. From the hinged position, swing the kettlebell back and behind your knees.

3. Swing the kettlebell up to shoulder level with your arms straight as you thrust your hips forward and raise your torso back into the standing position.

   • Make sure your butt muscles are engaged by squeezing your glutes together tightly.

   • Do not raise the kettlebell with your arms. Your arms and the kettlebell should feel weightless through the entire motion.

4. At the top of the swing, remember to keep your arms straight, and then thrust your hips forward, straighten your knees, and swing the kettlebell no higher than chest level as you rise to a standing position.

   • Do not bend back at the top of the motion.

5. Continue without stopping back down into your hinge and repeat steps 1–4. Create a nonstop fluid motion of the swing, with the kettlebell going behind the knees and back up to shoulder level.

MAKE IT A SINGLE-ARM SWING

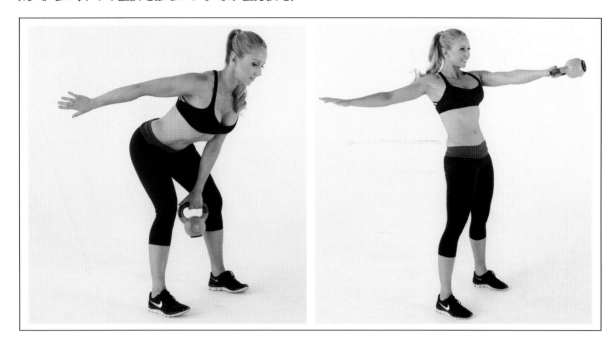

- You will be swinging the kettlebell with either your left or right arm.
- When you swing the kettlebell in one arm, make sure that as the kettlebell travels back and behind the legs, your thumb is facing back, not forward (this helps protect the elbow from hyperextension).
- Shoulder stability becomes more important with one arm, so keep your shoulder engaged and packed tight to your body.
- It is really important to engage the lats to prevent the shoulders from twisting.
- Think of the arm as a cable, merely holding the kettlebell with no tension.
- Do not try to lift the kettlebell with the arm; remember that this is a motion that engages your glutes and posterior chain, not the arms or quads.
- This is a single-side, single-arm swing, so stick to one side for the desired number or reps or time.

MAKE IT A SWING SWITCH

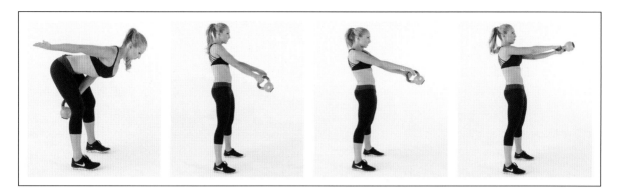

- Perform the exact same motion as described in your kettlebell swing, except now **switch** the kettlebell from one side to the other.
- Switch by bringing the other arm to meet and regrip the kettlebell.
- A good grip switch is to turn the palm up.
- Make sure to thrust your hips forward and engage your glutes at the top as you switch the kettlebell.

MAKE IT A DOUBLE KETTLEBELL SWING

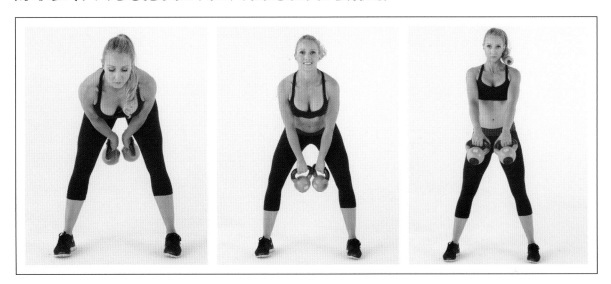

- Perform the exact same motion as described in the single-arm swing, except you will now be swinging two kettlebells instead of one.

- You may need to widen your stance in the legs to fit two kettlebells between your legs.

- Make sure to thrust your hips forward and engage your glutes at the top of the swing.

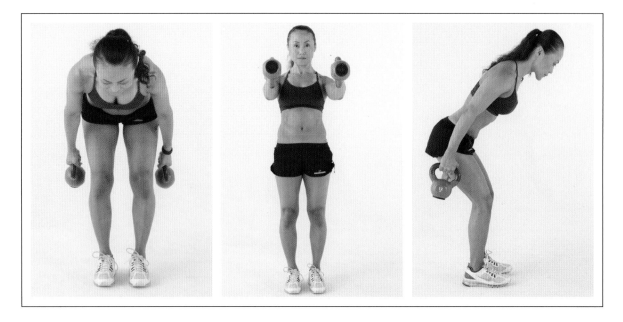

- The fundamental of the gun slinger swing is the standard double kettlebell swing, except now your kettlebells will be swung outside of the body.

- Take two kettlebells and place them at each side.

- Bring your feet together and make sure that they stay together the entire time.

- When you grip and pick up both kettlebells, make sure that your thumbs are facing forward and your palms are facing your legs.

- Take a hinge (exactly as illustrated in the kettlebell swing). Lead with the hips, and the knees will follow in a slight bend.

- Swing the kettlebells, keeping your core tight and your back strong and straight, aligning the spine head to hip.

- As both kettlebells reach shoulder level, squeeze your glutes, making sure not to backward bend, and bring the kettlebells back down.

MAKE IT A SUITCASE SWING

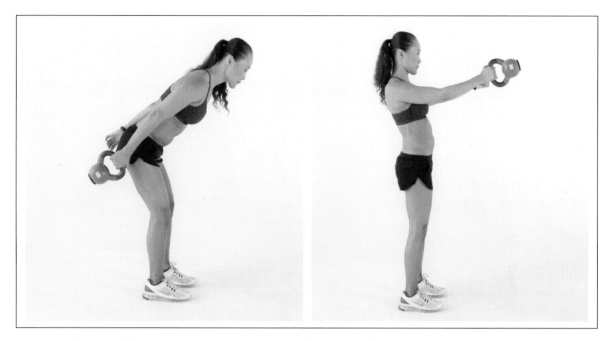

- This is the same exact motion as the gun slinger swing, except it is performed with only one kettlebell.
- Oddly this is more difficult than a double-handed swing because you will feel slightly off-balance due to the single-sided motion.
- Keep in mind that the fundamental of the suitcase swing is the standard kettlebell swing, except now your kettlebell will be swung outside of the body.
- Take one kettlebell and place it at your hip (on the same side as the hand that holds it).
- Bring your feet together and make sure that they stay together the entire time.
- When you grip and pick up the kettlebell, make sure that your thumb is facing forward and your palm is facing inward.
- Take a hinge (exactly as illustrated in the kettlebell swing). Lead with the hips, and the knees will follow in a slight bend.
- Swing the kettlebell, keeping your core tight and your back strong and straight, aligning the spine head to hip.
- As the kettlebell reaches shoulder level, squeeze your glutes, making sure not to backward bend, and bring the kettlebell back down.

Form

- Make sure you read chapter 4 to get the exact motion of the swing!

KB KICKS

Kicks work every single part of your body: the legs, the core, and yes—even the arms. However, we love how well these kicks train the glutes, and when paired with a kettlebell they are even better.

Snap Kick

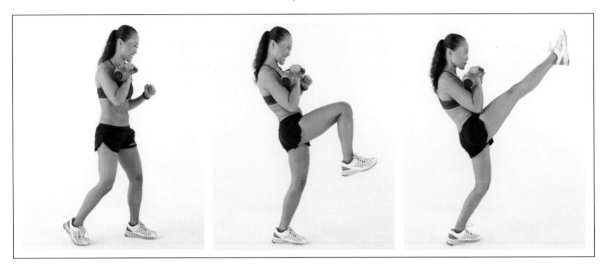

- Start from your boxing stance: lead leg forward and the rear leg on the ball of your foot, 90 degrees back.
- Bring up the rear leg and bend it at the knee.
- Snap the area between the knee and the ankle up, while pointing your toe.
- Return the leg back to your stance.
- You can alternate or continue with one leg.

Add a kettlebell to the motion if needed by holding the kettlebell in a racked position tight to the body.

Push Kick

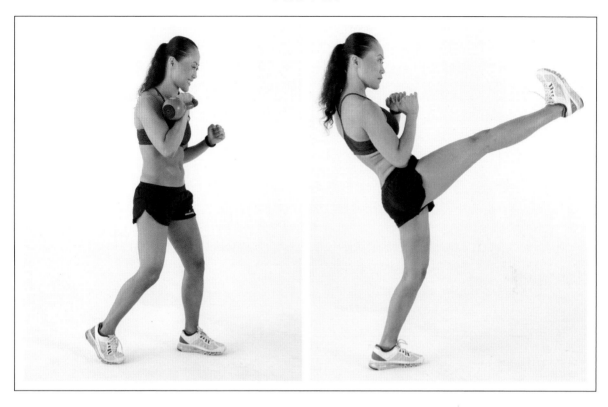

- Start from your boxing stance: lead leg forward and the rear leg on the ball of your foot, 90 degrees back.
- Bring up the rear leg and push it forward. Think about if you were trapped in a closet and had to get out by kicking down the door.
- Flex the foot straight out in front of you.
- Return the leg to your stance.
- You can alternate or continue with one leg.

Add a kettlebell to the motion if needed by holding the kettlebell in a racked position tight to the body.

Crescent Kick

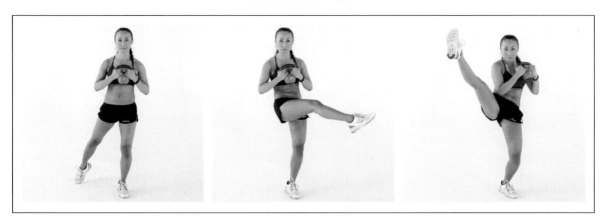

- Start from your boxing stance: lead leg forward and the rear leg on the ball of your foot, 90 degrees back.
- Bring up the rear leg and make a wide circle as you kick your leg around, inside to outside.
- Return the leg to your stance.
- You can alternate or continue with one leg.

Add a kettlebell to the motion if needed by holding the kettlebell in a racked position tight to the body.

Side Kick

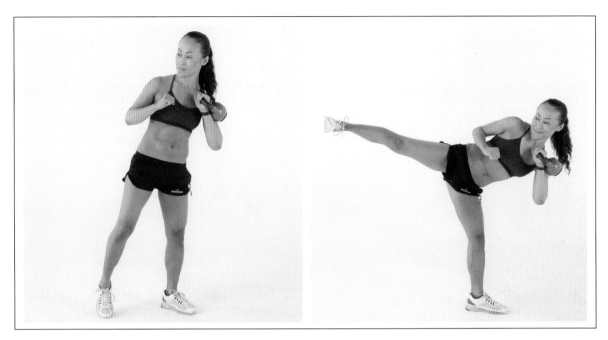

- Start from your boxing stance: lead leg forward and the rear leg on the ball of your foot, 90 degrees back.
- Bring up the rear leg and press it into the body.
- Then push your leg out to the side as you flex the foot straight out to the side of you.
- Return the leg to your stance.
- You can alternate or continue with one leg.

Add a kettlebell to the motion if needed by holding the kettlebell in a racked position tight to the body.

Donkey Kick

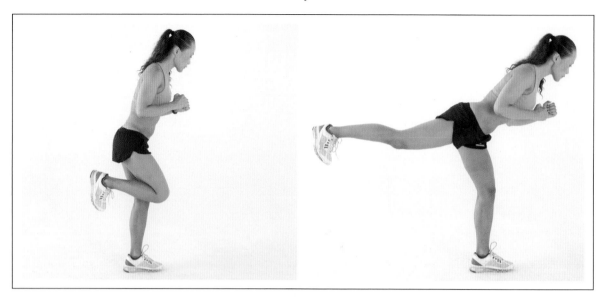

- Start from your boxing stance: lead leg forward and the rear leg on the ball of your foot, 90 degrees back.
- Bring up the rear leg and kick it back.
- Flex the foot of the kicking leg and use the power of your glutes.
- Snap the area between the knee and the ankle up, pointing your toe.
- Return the leg to your stance.
- You can alternate or continue with one leg.

Add a kettlebell to the motion if needed by holding the kettlebell in a racked position tight to the body.

DEAD LIFT

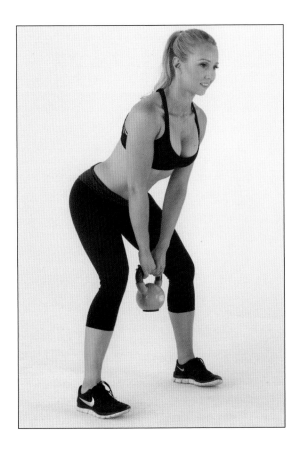

- Hold a kettlebell with an overhand grip by the handle; it should be hanging at arm's length in front of your hips, with no tension in the arms.

- Push your chest out.

- Keep your abdominals strong and your core tight and engaged.

- You will be doing a hinge, not a squat and not a stiff leg stretch.

- Set your feet hips' width apart.

- Hinge—hips go back first (bend at the hip) and then the knees bend slightly (you are not squatting).

- Without changing the bend in your knees, bend at your hips and lower your torso. It should feel like you are looking over a ledge.

- Then raise your torso back to the starting position.

- Do not round your lower back. The back should be straight, with a natural arch and packed shoulders.

- If executing with a kettlebell as illustrated, hold the kettlebell in front of you. Do not try to move it or push it out with your arms.

SINGLE-LEG (SL) DEAD LIFT

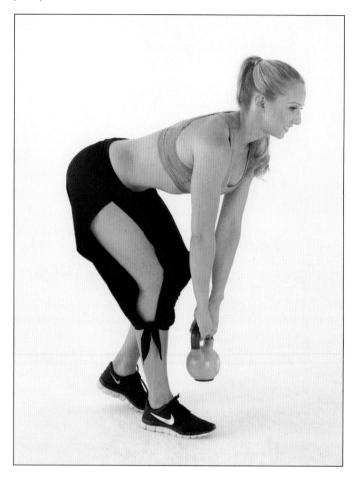

- Pick up the kettlebell with two hands and stand erect.
- Bend the right leg 90 degrees.
- Fold at the waist and sit back as the hips travel backward.
- Maintain a flat back, and on the inhale lower the kettlebell close to the ground.
- Exhale through the mouth and stand erect.
- The working leg bends slightly as you fold forward.
- The knees remain even throughout the exercise.

GOOD MORNING

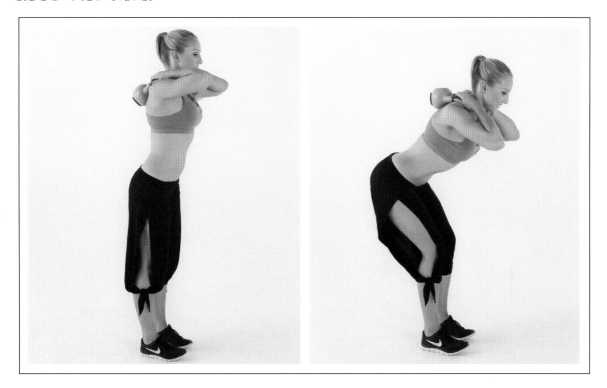

- Hold the kettlebell in a bottoms-up position by the horns.
- Use a half halo to bring the kettlebell back behind you.
- Place the kettlebell between the shoulder blades, behind you, and hold onto it.
- Feet are hips' width apart and parallel.
- Fold at the waist and bend forward in a hinge, not a squat.
- Keep the back arched and straight and the kettlebell behind you.
- You should be looking straight and in front of you; do not arch your neck up and out of alignment.

YO YO KB SQUAT

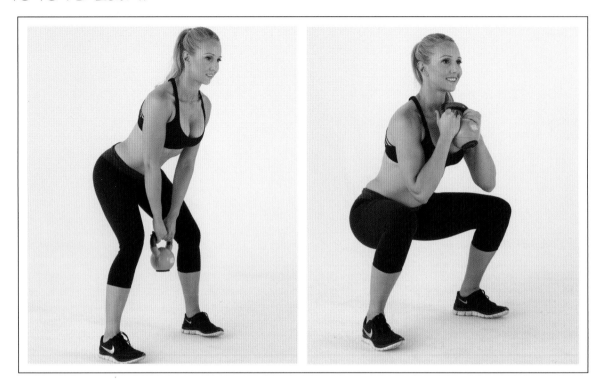

All squat and hinge forms you learned in chapters 4 and 7 apply!

- Hold the kettlebell by the handle, with your arms fully extended downward toward the ground.
- Your back should be straight and your shoulders pulled back.
- Start off with a hinge—like at the top of a dead lift or a kettlebell swing.
- Hinge down and reach the kettlebell toward the floor in a dead lift.
- Note: there should be a small bend in the knee, but no greater than the bend in your hip.
- As you come up from the dead lift, reach the kettlebell up and catch it with both hands by the horns; hold it in a mid-racked position.
- As you fix the kettlebell close to the body mid-racked, continue into a squat.
- As you come up from the squat, release your kettlebell from mid-racked to hanging position.
- You will be switching the kettlebell position as you switch between a hinge and a squat.

SPRAWL

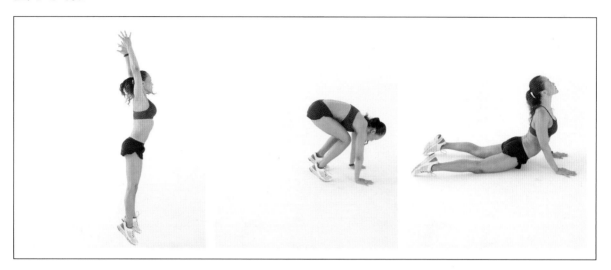

We placed this KB staple here because we love what the push up and back down does to the glutes. However, this is a complete, total-body motion that can be used to build and work any part of the body.

- Stand straight up and push off with your feet, using the power of the glutes by hinging back and up.
- Drop your body down to the floor.
- Arms should be extended as you press your chest away from the floor.
- Hips and legs and feet should be on the ground.
- Your feet should be open wide behind you, in a triangle.
- This looks a bit like, but is not, a burpee; unlike in the burpee, here you are not landing in a plank because your hips are touching the ground.
- Push your body back up to standing and repeat.

SNAP KICK TO SPRAWL

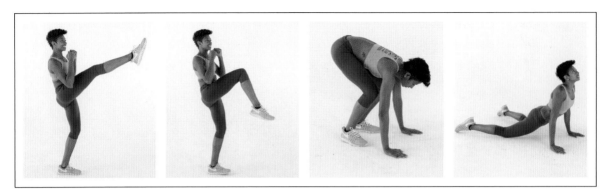

- You can add any of the kicks to your sprawl—we love the snap kick to sprawl combo.
- Just execute a snap kick after every sprawl.

BRIDGE

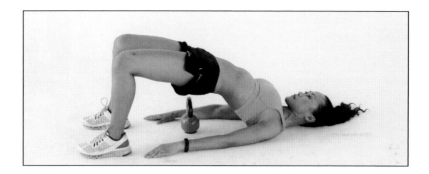

- Think of this as a hip raise or a reverse hinge.
- Lie faceup on the floor with your knees bent and your feet flat on the floor.
- Your heels should be pressed into the ground, while your toes can arch up off the ground.
- You should have all of your weight in your heels.
- Place your arms out to your sides.
- Raise your hips so your body forms a straight line from your shoulders to your knees.
- Continue to push against the floor with your heels, never your toes.
- Drive through your glutes as you lift your hips in a reverse hinge.
- Pause for a few seconds in the up position, then lower your body back down.

KB BRIDGE

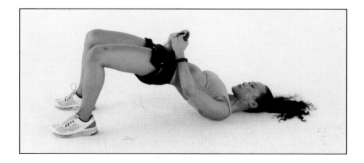

- Place a kettlebell on your hips and hold with both hands by the handle as you perform the same exercise as the bridge above.

SL KB BRIDGE

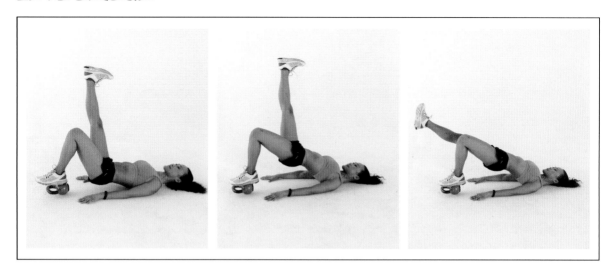

- Think of yourself as performing a single-leg hip raise.
- You can do this with or without a kettlebell placed on your hip.
- Lie faceup on the floor with one knee bent and your other leg straight out, elevated in front of you.
- Try to get your elevated leg in line with your thigh.
- Pressing through the heel of the stationary leg, push your hips upward, keeping your right leg elevated.
- Consider this a reverse hinge.
- Engage your glutes.
- Pause, and then slowly lower your body and leg back to the starting position.

Pictured here is a variation available to you by placing your foot on the belly of a kettlebell.

KB MERMAID

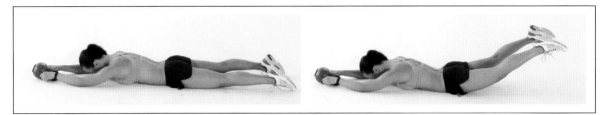

- Basically think of this as performing a reverse hip raise.
- Lie chest down on the floor or on the edge of a bench or Roman chair so that your torso is on the bench but your hips aren't.
- Lift your legs until your thighs are in line with your torso.
- Pause, then lower to the starting position.

FIRE HYDRANT

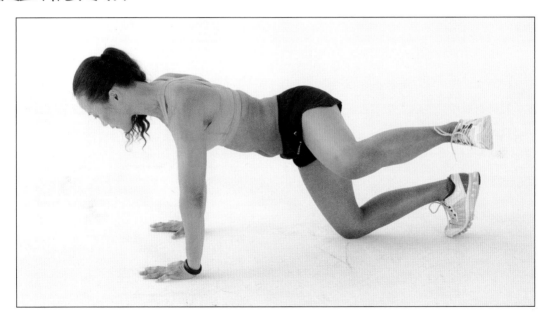

- Begin on all fours (hands and knees).
- Pick one leg and bend it at the knee.
- Then raise the leg up to hip level.
- Hold for a few seconds, keeping your core engaged and your glutes active.
- Switch to the other side or stay on one side.
- Complete 10–15 on each side or alternate for 1 minute per side.

ONE-INCH BUTT LIFTER

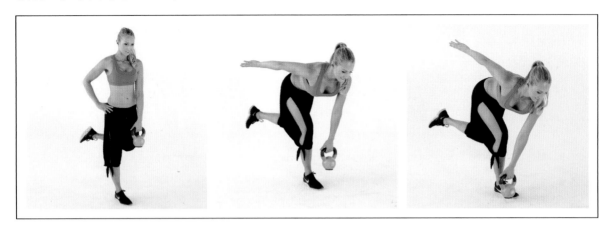

- Take a kettlebell, hold it by the handle in your left hand, and stand on your right foot with your knee slightly bent.
- Lift the left foot off of the floor and bend your knee slightly.
- Without changing the bend in your right knee, bend at your hips (hinge) and lower your torso as you rotate it to the right and touch the kettlebell to the floor past your right foot.
- Raise your torso back up.
- You should have all of your weight in the heel of the stationary foot and engage your glutes the entire time.
- Switch sides.

FOOT FIRE

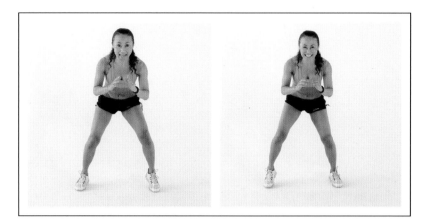

- Get in a stance with your feet slightly wider than your hips.
- Bend the knees slightly.
- Tighten your core and your glutes.
- Begin to move the feet quickly, as fast as you can.
- Every time you touch one foot to the floor, pick it up right away.
- Avoid any pressure on the knees.

SIDE SHUFFLES

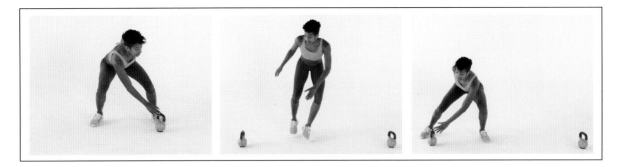

- Place two kettlebells 10 feet from one another.
- Get in a squat position.
- Shuffle side to side and touch the kettlebell on each side.
- Keep your back straight the entire time.

THE PERFECT BUTT WORKOUT PLAN

Here are some options for how to put everything together for your workout to achieve a great butt. They are in order from easiest to hardest.

For all workouts:
Start with 4–6 warm-up exercises from chapter 9.
End with 4–6 cool-down stretches from chapter 9.

Workout 1:

Complete 2 sets of any 8 exercises from this chapter in super sets of minute intervals.

Instead of doing the sets back to back and then going on to your next exercise, take your first 2 exercises and combine/alternate them. Do the same for the other 6 exercises, alternating exercises 3 and 4 for 2 sets each, and sets 5 and 6, and 7 and 8.

Work with a challenging weight/pace (depending on the move) that will leave you sweating for 1 minute of work/30 seconds of rest between each set.

Workout 2:

Complete 2 sets of any 8 exercises from this chapter.

However, instead of doing the sets back to back and then going on to your next exercise, take your first 2 exercises and combine/alternate them. Do the same for the other 6 exercises, alternating exercises 3 and 4 for 2 sets each, and sets 5 and 6, and 7 and 8.

Work with a challenging weight at 8–15 reps per move.
You should feel challenged, and you should max out at the weight.

Workout 3:

Complete 4 sets of any 4 exercises from this chapter.
Work with a challenging weight/pace (depending on the move) that will leave you sweating for 1 minute of work/30 seconds of rest between each.

Workout 4:

Complete 2 sets of any 8 exercises from this chapter.
Work with a challenging weight at 8–15 reps per move.
You should feel challenged, and you should max out at the weight.

Workout 5:

Run a circuit of 8 exercises from this chapter.
Complete one full rotation of all 8 exercises: 1 minute work and 30 seconds rest.
Repeat the circuit one more time, but this time do 1 minute work and 15 seconds rest.

Workout 6:

Pick 6 exercises from this chapter and place them into the following module:

- Perform the first and second exercises you picked for 8 rounds of 20 seconds of work and 10 seconds of rest for a total of 4 minutes of work.

- Rest for 2 minutes (a more advanced routine cuts this down to 1 minute of rest).

- Perform the third and fourth exercises you picked for 8 rounds of 20 seconds of work and 10 seconds of rest for a total of 4 minutes of work.

- Rest for 2 minutes (a more advanced routine cuts this down to 1 minute of rest).

- Perform the fifth and sixth exercises you picked for 8 rounds of 20 seconds of work and 10 seconds of rest for a total of 4 minutes of work.

- Rest for 2 minutes (a more advanced routine cuts this down to 1 minute of rest).

Use the move listed or any of the move's variations:

Box A	Box B	Box C
Use any move from chapters 4, 7, or 8.	Use any move from chapter 6.	Use any move from chapter 5.

Pick 3 exercises from the boxes on the previous page; one exercise from Box A, one from Box B, and one from Box C.

Place them into the following module:

- Perform the first exercise you picked for 8 rounds of 20 seconds of work and 10 seconds of rest for a total of 4 minutes of work.
- Rest for 2 minutes (a more advanced routine cuts this down to 1 minute of rest).
- Perform the second exercise you picked for 8 rounds of 20 seconds of work and 10 seconds of rest for a total of 4 minutes of work.
- Rest for 2 minutes (a more advanced routine cuts this down to 1 minute of rest).
- Perform the third exercise you picked for 8 rounds of 20 seconds of work and 10 seconds of rest for a total of 4 minutes of work.
- Rest for 2 minutes (a more advanced routine cuts this down to 1 minute of rest).
- Stretch using 3–6 stretches from chapter 9.

WARM-UPS, FLEXIBILITY, AND MOBILITY

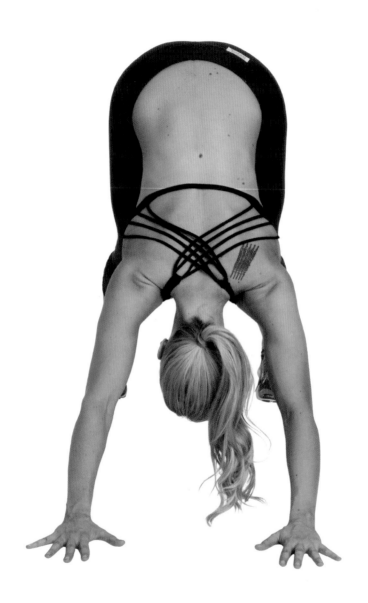

WARM UP AND COOL DOWN

Your workout is not complete without a good warm-up and cool-down. Think of them as the cornerstones of the workout. Make sure that you never skip this part of your training. In fact, do not consider it a workout unless you spent time both warming up (trust me—you'll perform better!) and cooling down (you will recover faster and be less likely to sustain injury from overuse or muscle imbalance). In your warm-up, we will work on taking your body through the same ranges found in your training; to do this we will be using dynamic stretching.

Dynamic Stretching—this form of stretching prepares the body for physical exertion and sports performance. Dynamic stretching increases range of movement, as well as blood and oxygen flow to soft tissues prior to exertion. Dynamic stretches are fast yet controlled. They typically last no longer than 2–3 seconds. How is it done? This is your warm-up! It progressively takes the body through all of the ranges of motion you will encounter in your training routine.

In your cool-down, we will hold our stretch through a prolonged period of time, creating actual change in the length of the muscle.

Static Stretching—this is used to stretch muscles and muscle groups while the body is at rest. In Kettlebell Kickboxing, we do this after the workout is complete. Static stretching is composed of various techniques that gradually lengthen a muscle to an elongated position (to the point of slight discomfort); we hold that position for 30 seconds to 2 minutes. The minimum duration to get the benefits of stretching is 30 seconds, whereas 2 minutes is the standard maximum (if a position can be held for more than 2 minutes, a further stretch should be performed).

Do not skip over these parts of the workout; the warm-up and cool-down portions are just as important as any other part of your workout. Pick and execute your warm-up and cool-down exercises from the illustrated step-by-steps that follow, and make sure to include them in every KB session.

> **Recent studies show that traditional static stretching techniques do little to increase flexibility or reduce injury when performed before a workout, but can significantly enhance performance and minimize injury and sore muscles when done after a workout. Keep static stretching at the end of your KB workout.**

Let's look at warm-up options!

MOBILITY is most important!

Mobility is the single most defining and important factor in your fitness. It is not strength or flexibility that matters most— it is mobility. What is mobility? By a basic definition, it is the ability to move freely; in the fitness world, we would define this as the area where your strength and flexibility meet.

A visual example would be if I hold your leg up as high as your body allowed—that would be your flexibility. Your strength alone would be how much weight that leg can lift or push in a strength-based motion like a squat or lunge. But your mobility is the ability and height of that leg when you hold it up, using both flexibility and strength together (with no aid from anyone else).

This is important because in fitness, mobility is true health! Remember that your body can't *just* be strong or *just* be flexible; the two are not complete without each other. Working toward mobility is working toward pain-free movement and the freedom to use your body at its best capacity.

How do you work your mobility? The Kettlebell Kickboxing workout is full of drills that develop mobility. Just about every kick and swing you do will help develop that for you. Another way to help develop mobility is in your warm-ups and cool-downs.

LET'S WARM UP

A warm-up should be between 5 to 10 minutes in length, depending on how stiff you feel. Traditionally your warm-ups should take you through all of the ranges of motion you will encounter in your training. For us, that includes kicks, planks, light locomotion, and other forms of body activation.

For any of your workouts in this book, or even in general, you will start by picking three to six motions and then execute them for time, ideally 1 minute each. After you have finished your warm-up, continue straight into the prescribed exercises. Do not static stretch until the end of your workout.

ADVANCED: 2-minute stationary run

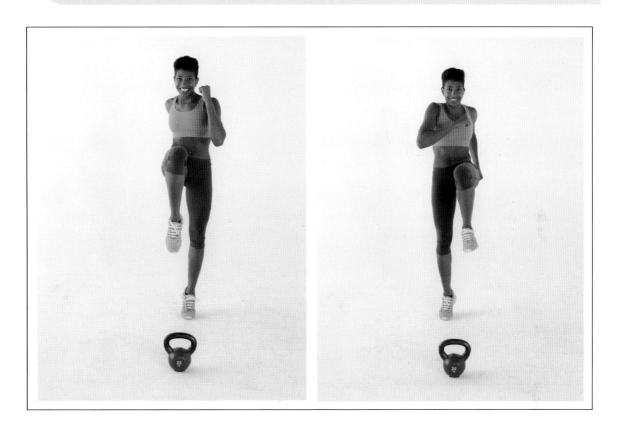

- I know it seems simple, but running at a steady pace for 1 minute is tough. And for 2 minutes—really tough!
- Place a kettlebell in front of you for a reference point of how high your feet should come up in the run.
- Step away from the kettlebell and begin to run in place; your feet should never come lower than the kettlebell handle.
- Aim for 2 minutes as an awesome warm-up to any activity.
- Do not try to touch the kettlebell with your feet.
- Do not slow down, and do not let your feet drag.
- Use your arms to help you run.

SKIPPING

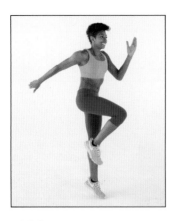

- It seems funny, but skipping is one of the most natural ways to warm up the body.
- Your body will recognize the skipping motion because you have done it since you were a child.
- Try a minute of stationary or moving skips.
- Keep the pressure off of the joints and skip naturally, landing lightly.

HOPS

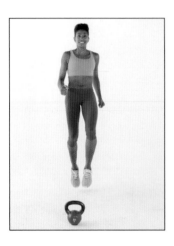

- Place the kettlebell in front of you for a reference point.
- Step away from the kettlebell.
- Begin to hop very lightly and with good form.
- Abdominals should be tight and glutes engaged.
- Make sure in every hop, you hop as high as the kettlebell handle.
- Work nonstop for 1 minute.
- Always land lightly.

BOB AND WEAVE (NO KETTLEBELL)

- Take a kickboxing stance with one leg forward and the other about 90 degrees behind.
- Place the weight on the ball of your rear foot and twist down a little and toward your front foot as if you are ducking a punch coming at you from your rear foot's side.
- Dip down in a mini squat and make a small half circle with your head as you come up, slightly shifting the head.
- Keep the arm bent and tight to the body.
- Switch directions, coming back through a mini squat/dip to the starting position.
- Do not forget to switch your stance for the next set.
- Work nonstop for 1 minute.

USE YOUR JAB-CROSS COMBOS

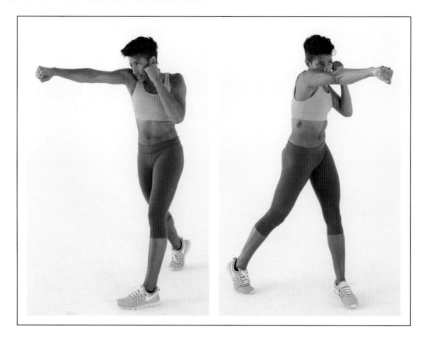

- Use the jab-cross combinations and form described in chapter 6 to warm up the arms, upper body, and spine.
- Perform the combo in your right lead for 1 minute.
- Then switch to the left lead for another minute.

DEEP SQUAT WARM-UP

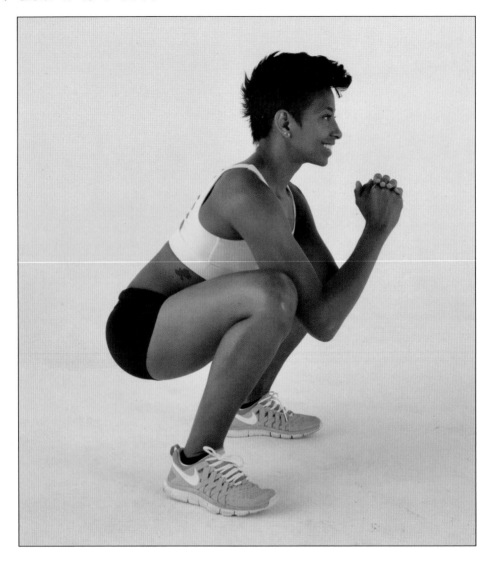

- Use the exact same squat form and step-by-step as we illustrated in chapter 7.

- Execute deep and very controlled squats without weight.

- Make sure that there is no pressure on the joints, and do not rush.

- Engage the glutes, legs, and abdominals.

- Do 15 squats or work for 1 minute.

OVERHEAD WARM-UP SQUAT

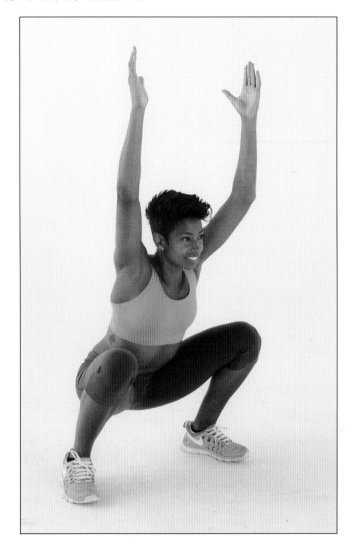

- Use the same form and motion as was illustrated in the overhead squat step-by-step in chapter 7.
- For the warm-up, use no kettlebell.
- This is still an advanced motion.
- Take your time.
- Perform 5–10 reps or a 1-minute warm-up set.

SINGLE-ARM OVERHEAD REACHES

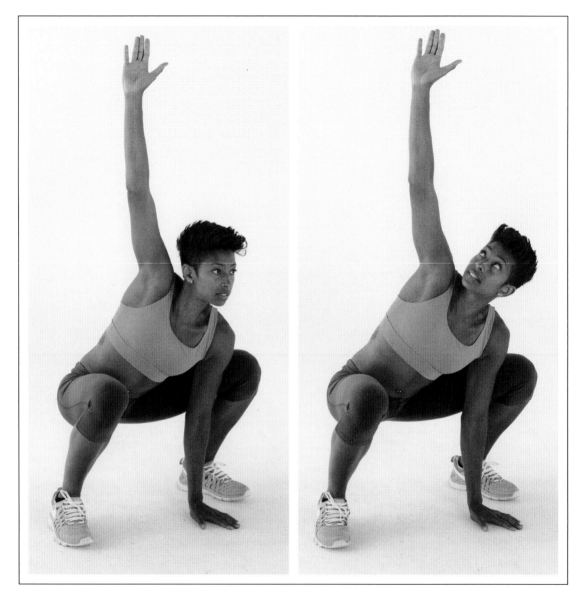

- As you squat down, reach down and touch the floor with one arm.
- Reach the opposite arm overhead.
- Alternate sides and follow all squat form.
- Alternate for 1 minute straight, or work for 10 reps on each side.
- It is easier to look up at the arm; looking forward is more challenging. Try to work your way to doing both with comfort.

MID-BACK ACTIVATION

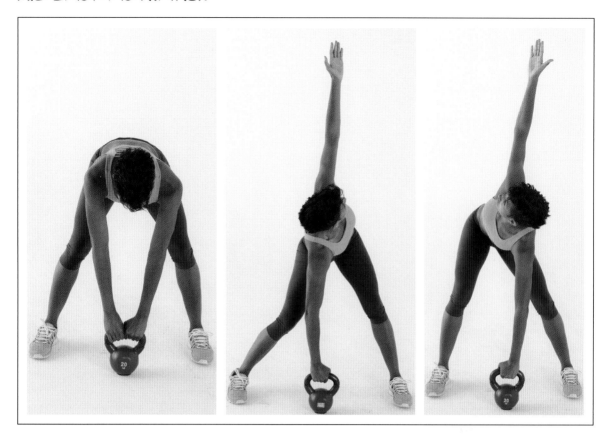

A must if you sit most of your day.

- Place a kettlebell on the ground and place both hands on its handle.
- Hinge over the kettlebell and make sure that your back is straight from the hip to the neck.
- Raise one arm up and look up, but do not move the rest of your body.
- Your job is to activate your mid-back.
- Get your arm as high and far behind you as possible.
- Repeat on the other side.
- Alternate for 10 slow reps per side.

LIGHT JUMPS

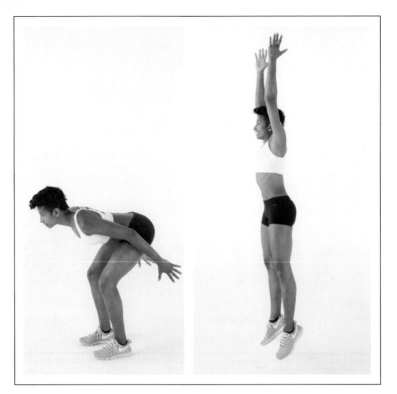

- You can use jumping for a warm-up; however, you must follow proper form.
- Each jump should be executed from a hinge, so that the glutes can be engaged.
- Do not pound on the knees or go too fast.
- Go slow and take your time, activating and warming up the body.
- Try 10–15 controlled jumps or 1 minute of work.

KICKING WARM-UPS

- You can use any of the kicks detailed in chapter 8 to warm up the body.
- You can alternate each kick or stick to one side.
- Do not add weights or kettlebells.
- Execute each kick for 1 minute on each side, or alternating sides.
- You can also combine the kicks (snap-push-crescent kick combos, in any combination).

Reach Kick

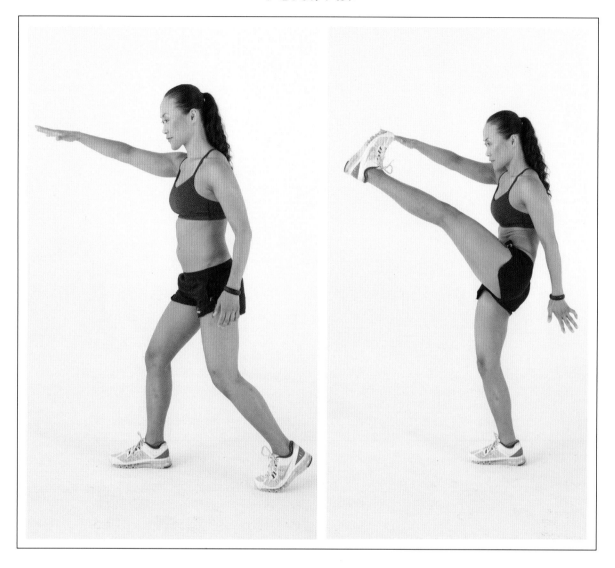

- Start from your boxing stance: lead leg forward and the rear leg on the ball of your foot, 90 degrees back.

- Bring the rear leg straight up, as if you were kicking up a soccer ball.

- Kick the leg up as high as you can and reach the opposite side arm to touch the foot.

- Return the leg back to your stance.

- You can alternate or continue with one leg.

Snap Kick

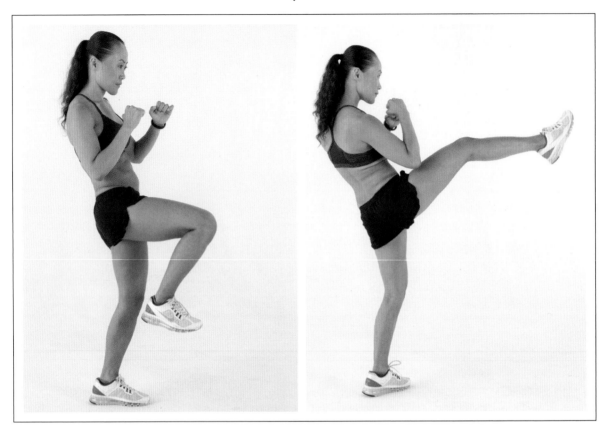

- Start from your boxing stance: lead leg forward and the rear leg on the ball of your foot, 90 degrees back.

- Bring up the rear leg and bend it at the knee.

- Snap the area between the knee and the ankle up, pointing your toe.

- Return the leg back to your stance.

- You can alternate or continue with one leg.

Push Kick

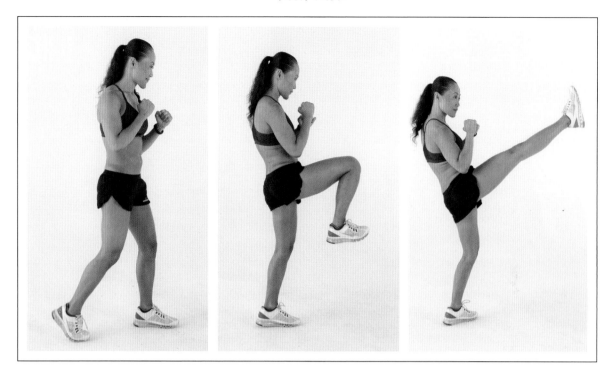

- Start from your boxing stance: lead leg forward and the rear leg on the ball of your foot, 90 degrees back.
- Bring up the rear leg and push it forward.
- Flex the foot straight out in front of you.
- Return the leg back to your stance.
- You can alternate or continue with one leg.

Side Kick

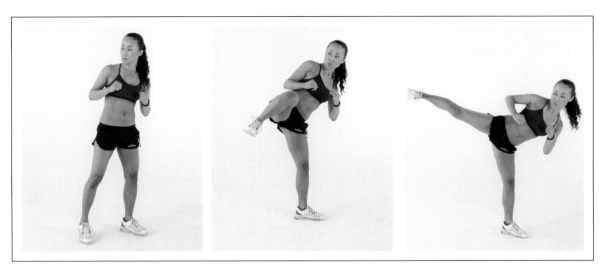

- Start from your boxing stance: lead leg forward and the rear leg on the ball of your foot, 90 degrees back.
- Bring up the rear leg and press it into the body.
- Then push your leg out to the side as you flex the foot straight out to the side of you.
- Return the leg to your stance.
- You can alternate or continue with one leg.

Crescent Kick

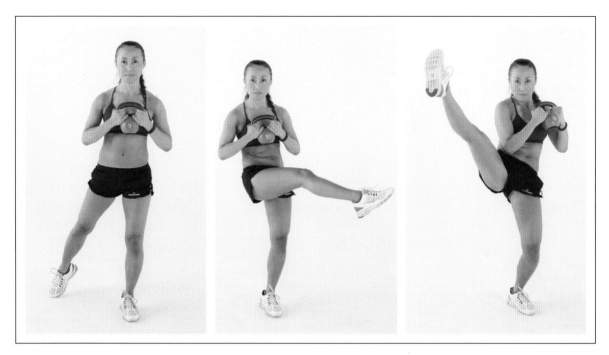

- Start from your boxing stance: lead leg forward and the rear leg on the ball of your foot, 90 degrees back.

- Bring up the rear leg and make a wide circle as you kick your leg around, inside to outside.

- Return the leg to your stance.

- You can alternate or continue with one leg.

Donkey Kick

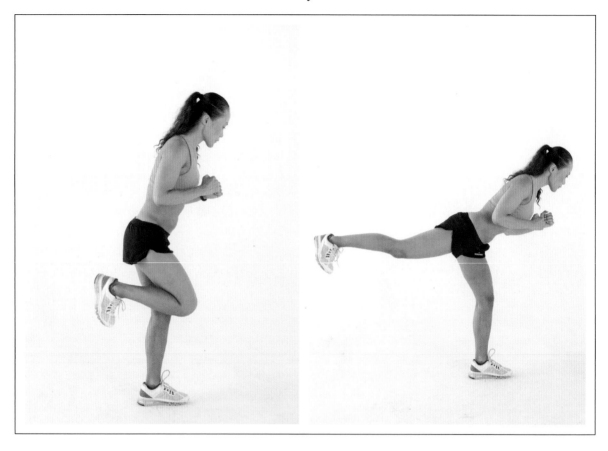

- Start from your boxing stance: lead leg forward and the rear leg on the ball of your foot, 90 degrees back.
- Bring up the rear leg and kick it back.
- Flex the foot of the kicking leg and use the power of your glutes.
- Snap the area between the knee and the ankle up, pointing your toe.
- Return the leg to your stance.
- You can alternate or continue with one leg.

PLANK TO DOWNWARD DOG

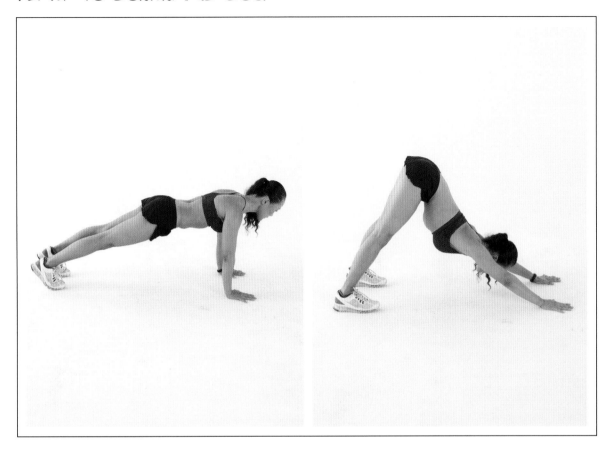

- Starting off in a good plank position, begin to bring your hips up to the sky.
- As you shift your hips, press your shoulder blades together.
- Try to straighten your legs as much as you can, and try to touch your heels to the ground (only if you can).
- You should have an equal amount of your weight distributed between the legs and arms.

CATERPILLAR

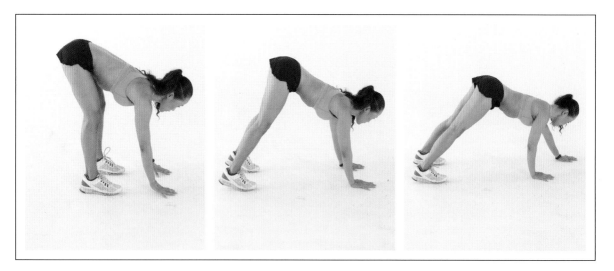

- From standing, walk out slowly and with control into a plank.
- Stay in plank for just a moment, and then continue to walk back up.
- Use your full body and make sure that you feel a good stretch in the back of the legs, arms, and back as you walk out and back.
- Continue for 10–15 reps or 1 minute of work.

SPIDER STRETCH

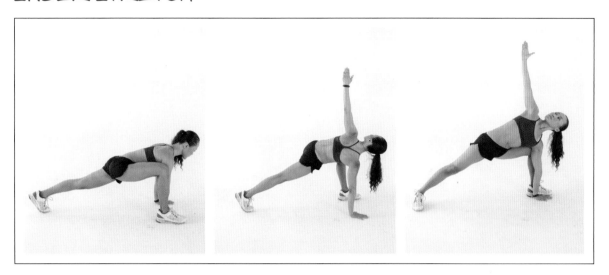

- Starting in a plank, jump or step one leg up by the outside of both arms.
- Note that you should eventually have the mobility to bring the leg that far—maybe you can't yet, but over time you should.
- As you step your foot forward, reach the outside arm up to the sky and look up. Plant on the ground the arm that is on the opposite side as the front foot.
- Then switch your arms (leaving the legs as they are) and reach the opposite arm up and look up.
- Then step back into the plank and switch sides for the legs.
- Continue for 1 minute.

WINDMILL ROTATION

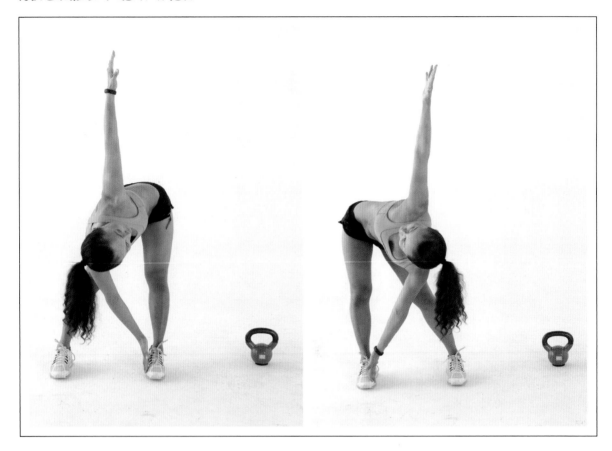

- Begin by standing with your legs slightly wider than the hips.
- Keeping the legs as straight as possible, reach the opposite arm to the opposite leg.
- Keep the opposite arm up and look up toward it.
- Alternate sides, but as you go to switch, pause in the center, stand, and then go to the other side.
- Also pause at each side of the stretch.

FINGER PUSH-UPS

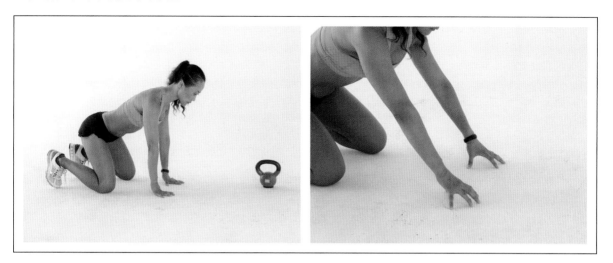

- Get on all fours (hands and knees) and place both palms out in front of you.
- Now push off of your palms onto your fingers and back down in a very slow and controlled pace.
- Make sure you feel every part of the motion in your wrists, palms, and fingers.

COOL-DOWN TIME!

Cool-down is your time to stretch the muscles. After a workout, the muscles are warm and mobile and should be more receptive to slower, longer, and deeper static stretching. Traditionally, static stretching should be done on a warm body. This helps prevent injury and gets you into a deeper, safer stretch. Cooling down will also help you recover faster, and help you work on the very important length-tension relationships.

- Perform **at least** two exercises from each area of the body after your Kettlebell Kickboxing workout. Ideally you should do three to four from the two areas listed: upper and lower.

- Hold the stretches for at least 25 seconds, and ideally between 45 seconds to 1 minute; however, if your body is telling you that you need to hold the stretch longer, then listen to it and do so. Do not skip this portion of the program!

MAIN FOCUS: LOWER BODY

STANDING HAMSTRING STRETCH

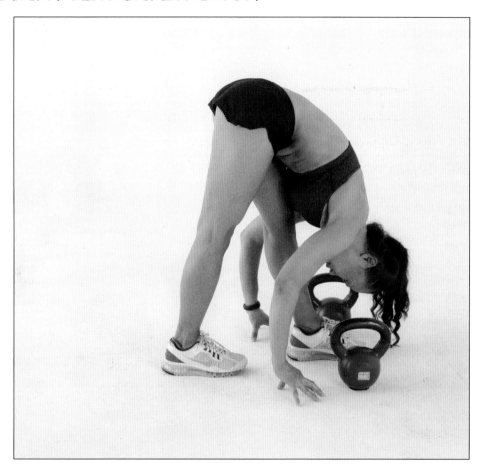

- Step one foot on the floor in front of you, with both legs completely straight.
- Stand tall with your back naturally arched.
- Slightly bend the front leg at the knee.
- Reach your hands down to the ground.
- If you cannot reach the ground yet, place two kettlebells at each side and reach toward them.
- Your hips should be aligned and your neck relaxed and not arching up.
- Try to bring your forehead to the knee and fold your body to your front leg.
- Continue to try to get deeper into the stretch on every exhale.

SITTING HAMSTRING STRETCH

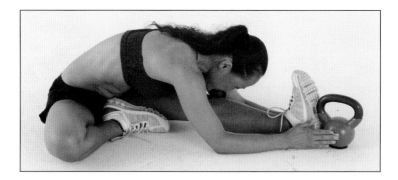

- Sit down on the ground and bring one leg out in front of you as you bend the other one in.
- Fold your body down and try to reach your forehead to your knee.
- On the exhale, aim to stretch the leg out fully.

KB SITTING HAMSTRING STRETCH

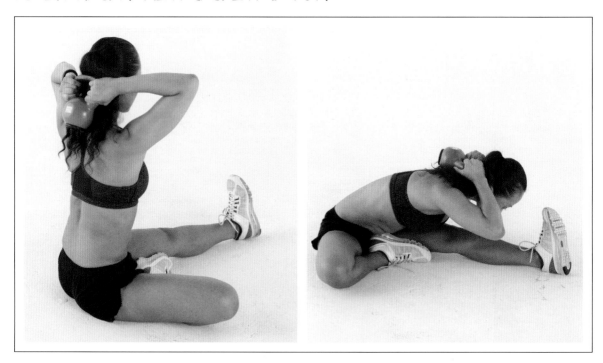

- Use a kettlebell to help you get deeper into the stretch as shown above, but only if you are comfortable with the kettlebell.

SIDE SPLIT STRETCH

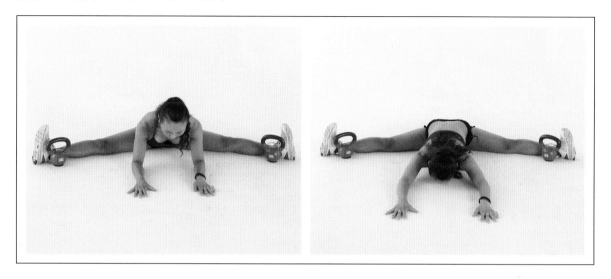

- Use the kettlebells to help you keep both legs in a side split position.
- Reach down with both arms and walk yourself out, getting your chest as close to the ground as possible.
- Continue to try to get deeper into the stretch on every exhale.

KB SIDE SPLIT STRETCH

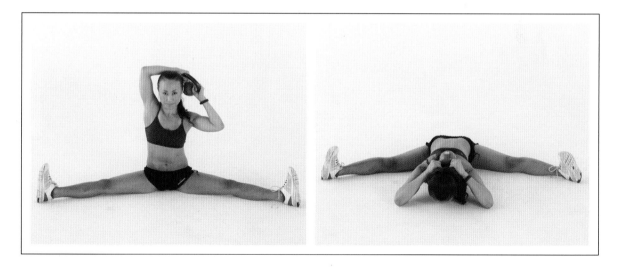

- Only if you're comfortable, use the kettlebell behind you as pictured to help you get deeper into the stretch.

RUNNER LUNGE

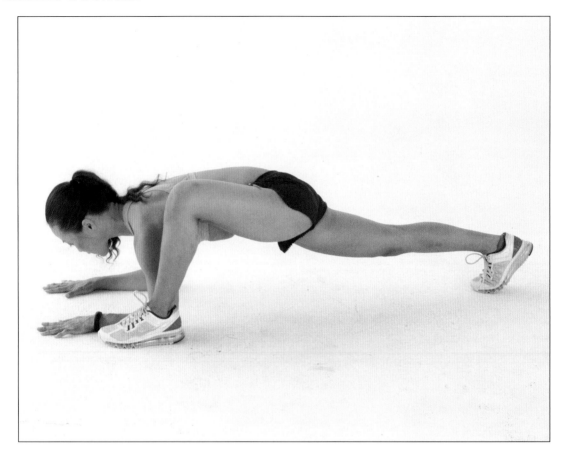

- Get into a plank and bring one foot up to meet the arm on the same side, on the outside of the arm.
- Then try to bring both elbows down to the ground through the exhale.

STANDING QUAD STRETCH

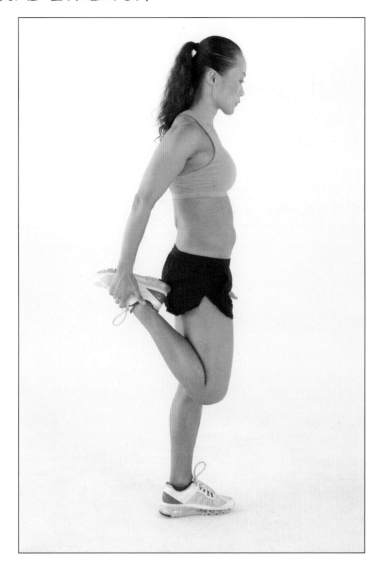

- While standing, bring one leg back and bend it at the knee.
- Hold the foot with the arm on the same side (grasping the outside of the foot), and as you engage your glutes, gently assist by pulling the leg back.
- You should feel a stretch in the front of the leg.
- You can use a wall for balance.
- Do not overpull the leg; instead, engage your glutes to get a deeper stretch.

FRONT SPLIT STRETCH

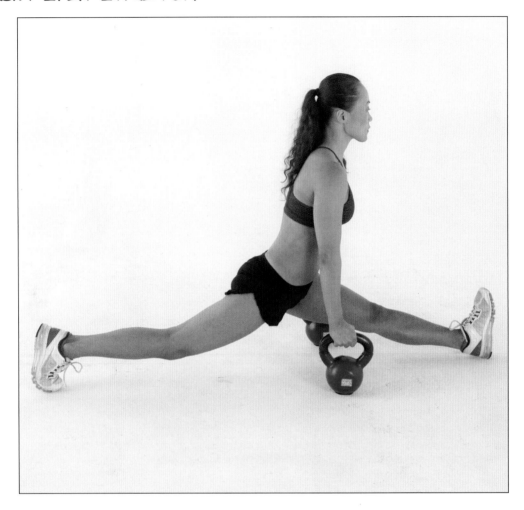

- You should use two large kettlebells for stability.
- As you aim to complete a front split, use the kettlebells to help you ease into the posture.
- You must keep your core engaged to maintain stability.
- On the exhale, try to get deeper and deeper into the stretch.

HURDLE STRETCH

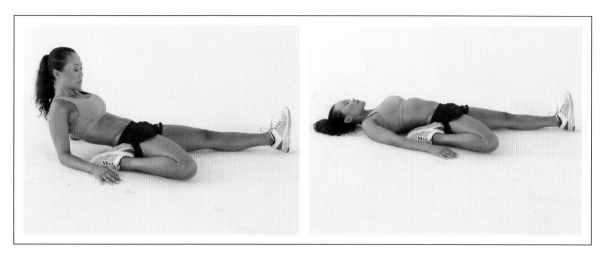

- Sit back and stretch one leg out in front of you.
- Bend the other leg back behind you (bending at the knee).
- If you can lay your torso all the way back, do so, but do not force it.
- Make sure you do not rush into this stretch. You should never feel any pressure on the knee; if you do, do the standing quad stretch instead.

YOGI STRETCH

- Bring both feet together as pictured below, but do not cross them.
- Begin to lower your body down, starting with your chest.
- Keep your back straight the entire time.
- Keep your neck neutral and do not arch it up.
- Try to get even deeper into the stretch on the exhale.

KETTLEBELL YOGI STRETCH

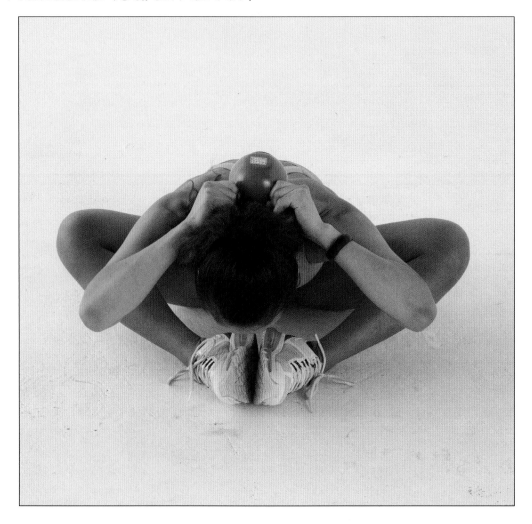

- Complete the same exact stretch as we just saw, except place a kettlebell behind your back to help you get deeper into the motion.

GLUTE AND HAMSTRING STRETCH

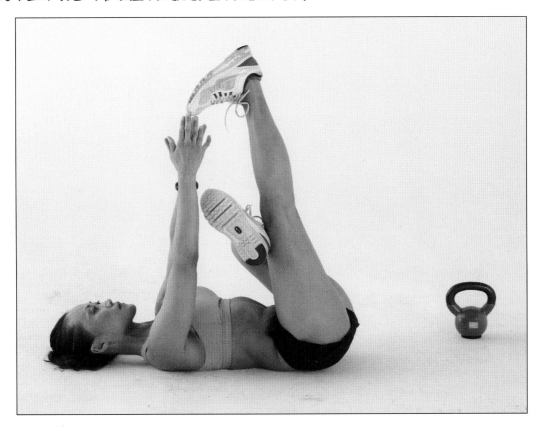

- Lie on your back and bring one foot up, fully extended out in front of you.
- Bend and hook the opposite leg inside the extended foot, as pictured.
- Begin to pull the extended leg into the body, keeping it straight.
- You should feel a deep hamstring stretch in the extended leg and a glute stretch in the bent leg.

GLUTE STRETCH

- From a seated position, bend one leg in as you hold the other leg right on top of it.
- Begin to lower your body down, starting with your chest.
- Keep your back straight the entire time.
- Keep your neck neutral and do not arch it up.
- Try to get even deeper on the exhale.

KETTLEBELL GLUTE STRETCH

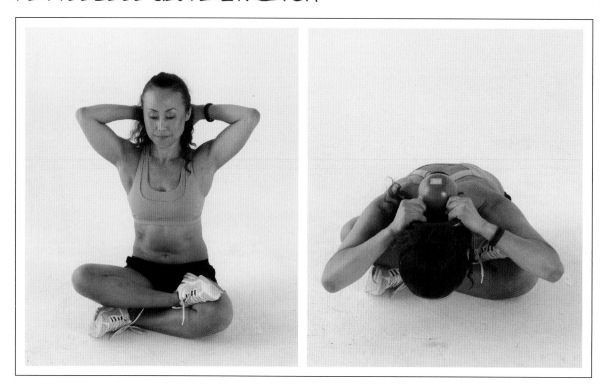

- Complete the glute stretch, except place a kettlebell behind your back to help you get deeper into the motion.

TOE STRETCH

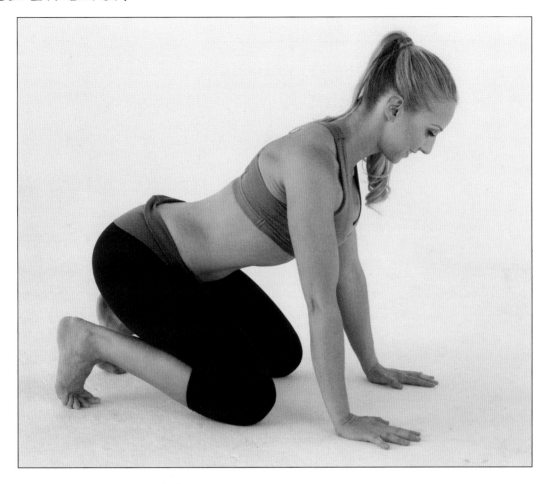

- Sit back on your knees and curl the toes onto the ground.
- Make sure that your shoes are off.
- Slowly sit back deeper, getting mobility in the toes.
- Eventually this should begin to feel comfortable.

MAIN FOCUS: UPPER BODY

WALL STRETCH

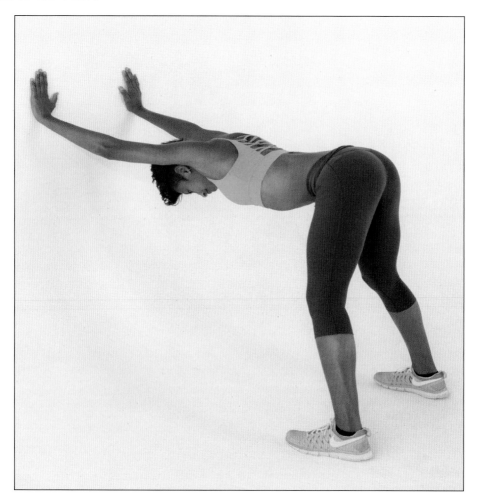

- Place both your palms on a wall in front of you and walk back as you begin to lean forward.
- You should feel a deep lat stretch as well as a nice stretch throughout the arms, chest, shoulder, and back.
- Keep your neck neutral and do not arch it up.

KNEELING LAT STRETCH

- Kneel on the floor and place your kettlebell a few feet in front of you, placing your hands on the kettlebell handle.
- Lean forward at your hips and press your shoulders toward the floor, maintaining a small arch in the back and keeping arms off of the floor.

LAT AND ARM STRETCH

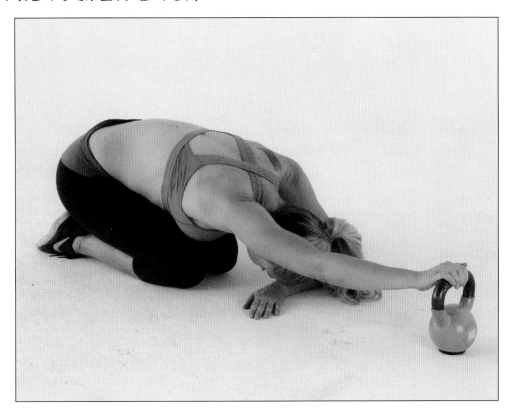

- Place a kettlebell in front of you as you sit on your knees and lean forward.
- Reach one arm out and place it on the handle of the standing kettlebell.
- Sit back and do not let the arm touch the ground.
- Reach and breathe, feeling a deep stretch in your back and arms.
- Your neck should be relaxed and neutral.
- You can also cushion your head with your other arm.

WRIST STRETCH

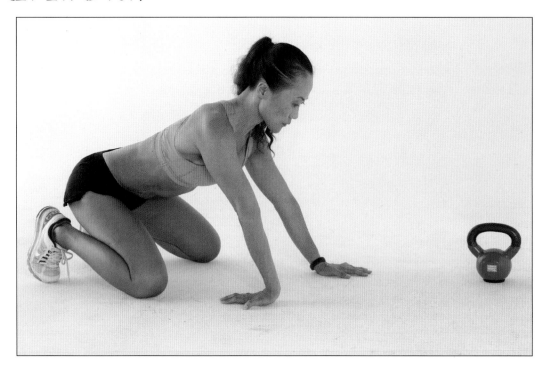

- Get on all fours and bring both arms out in front of you.
- Place one arm on the floor with the hand facing forward, palm on the ground.
- Place the other arm with the palm facing you, and try to reach that palm to the ground.
- To get deeper into the stretch, sit your butt back and down onto your heels.
- Alternate sides.

DOWNWARD DOG

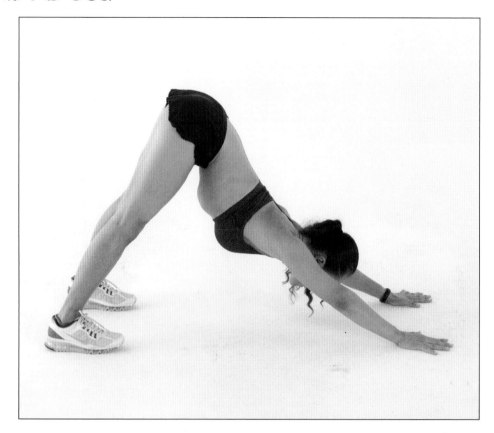

- The downward dog can be used as a total-body activation and stretch.
- The back and arms should feel like they are being activated and mobilized.
- The legs, including calves and hamstrings, should also feel a deep stretch.
- Starting off in a good plank position, begin to bring your hips up to the sky.
- As you shift your hips, press your shoulder blades together.
- Try to straighten your legs as much as you can, and try to touch your heels to the ground (only if you can).
- You should have equal amount of weight distributed between the legs and arms.

KB SHOULDER AND CHEST STRETCH

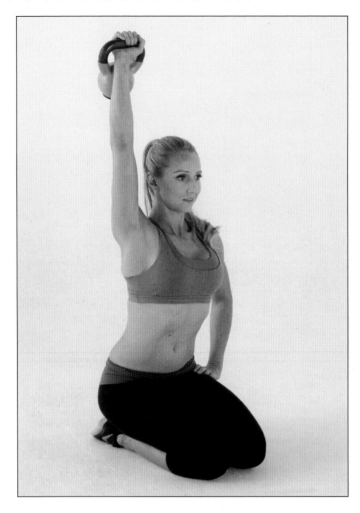

- Sit on your knees comfortably.
- Bring one kettlebell of a light weight overhead and allow it to stretch your shoulder and your chest.
- Make sure to keep the shoulder packed and secure.
- You should not have any shoulder injuries if you choose to do this stretch.

SHOULDER STRETCH

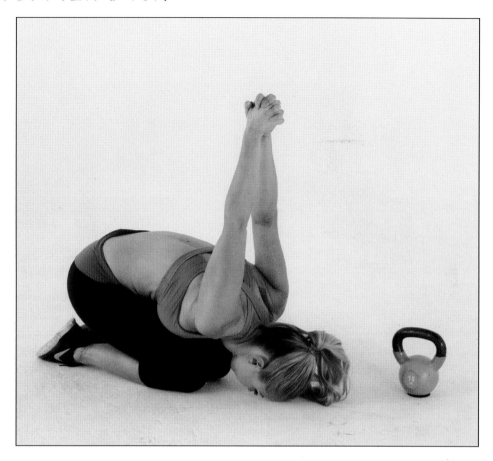

- Sit on your knees, lean forward, and reach both arms out behind your back.
- Clench the palms together and squeeze them together.
- You should feel a deep shoulder stretch.
- You should aim to have enough mobility to have the palms touch, but you may not be able to at first if you have tight shoulders.

COBRA STRETCH

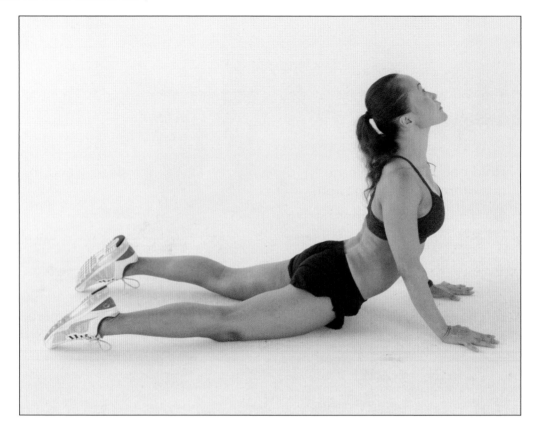

- Lie down on your stomach. Pull your shoulder blades back as you press your upper body off of the ground with both arms.

- Do not overarch the back.

- Instead, just look up and feel a deep stretch in the back, arms, shoulders, and neck.

- Keep your glutes engaged the entire time.

FEELING TIGHT?

If you are feeling tight, do a Kettlebell Kickboxing recovery workout!

Try This KB Recovery Workout:

- Start off with any 6 warm-up moves and rotate them twice for 1 minute each.
- Don't take a break in between the warm-up motions; just flow.
- Continue on to 5 lower body stretches.
- Hold each for 1–2 minutes and make sure to breathe deeply and try to relax through each motion.
- Continue on to 5 upper body stretches.
- Hold each motion between 45 seconds to 1 minute and make sure to breathe deeply and try to relax through each motion.

BONUS! Want to add some sweat?
- After your warm-up, pick up a kettlebell and do 4 rounds of 1-minute swings, resting for 15–30 seconds between each set.
- Then move on to a cool-down.

CHAPTER 10

BURN 500

Burn up to 500 Calories in 30 Minutes or Less!

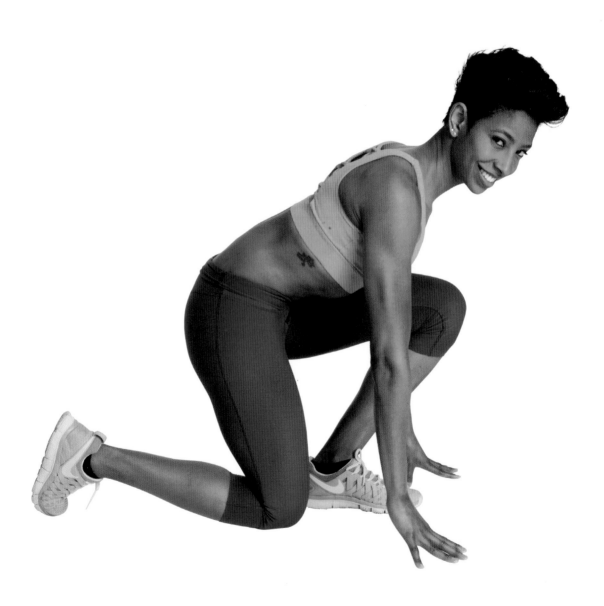

This chapter arranges a great variety of motions from chapters 5–8 to help you efficiently burn 500 calories in one session. The following chapter (11) will use time intervals to make the most out of these **Burn 500** workouts.

I would love for you to consider these motions as a series of poses and moves that fully utilize the power and strength of your body. Connecting KB exercises creates a soothing flow that promotes endurance. Instead of the stop-and-go motion of a squat or a lunge, the movements should come together, smoothly **flowing** and almost dance-like. However, you cannot forget to give your full attention to each motion separately, with emphasis on both form and transitioning between reps and sets.

Your KB Burn 500 workout flows are listed in this chapter. **Your goal in the Burn 500 workout?** Combine three flows and execute them for a complete Burn 500 workout. If you are short on time, you can also execute just one or two flows.

- Before your first flow, spend 3–5 minutes performing a light warm-up using 3–5 warm-ups from chapter 9.
- At the end of your last flow, spend 5–10 minutes performing 3–5 cool-down stretches from chapter 9.
- Please note that the form and step-by-step pictures of each exercise are discussed in chapters 5 through 8.
- You should be comfortable with each base move of the flow before you move on to the flow itself. The base motion is in the title of each flow.

BURN 500 FLOW: KB SWING FLOWS

KB Flow 1

Set one:
- Perform 1 KB swing.
- Catch the kettlebell to mid-racked position.
- Continue on to a squat.
- Press the kettlebell overhead at the top of the squat.
- Bring the kettlebell back to mid-racked position.
- Slowly slide the kettlebell back to hanging and start again.

After that . . .
- Set two: perform 2 kettlebell swings and 2 squats.
- Set three: perform 3 kettlebell swings and 3 squats.
- Continue to 25 reps of swings and 25 squats in between the two motions.

KB Flow 2

Set one:
- Perform 1 KB swing.
- Catch the kettlebell to mid-racked position.
- Continue on to alternating rear lunges.
- As you come back out of each lunge, perform a push kick forward.
- Press the kettlebell overhead.
- Bring the kettlebell back to mid-racked position.
- Slowly slide the kettlebell back to hanging and start again.

After that . . .
- Set two: perform 2 kettlebell swings and 2 lunges.
- Set three: perform 3 kettlebell swings and 3 lunges.
- Continue to 26 reps of swings and 26 lunges (13 on each leg) in between the two motions.

KB Flow 3

Set one:
- Perform a gun slinger swing.
- Clean the kettlebells to mid-racked position.
- Continue on to a squat.
- Press the kettlebells overhead at the top of the squat.
- Bring the kettlebells back to mid-racked position.
- Slowly slide the kettlebells back to hanging and start again.

After that . . .
- Set two: perform 2 gun slinger swings and 2 squats.
- Set three: perform 3 gun slinger swings and 3 squats.
- Continue to 25 reps of swings and 25 squats in between the two motions.

KB Flow 4

Set one:
- Perform a double KB high pull swing.
- Clean the kettlebells to mid-racked position.
- Continue on to a squat.
- Press the kettlebells overhead at the top of the squat.
- Bring the kettlebells back to mid-racked position.
- Slowly slide the kettlebells back to hanging and start again.

After that . . .
- Set two: perform 2 kettlebell high pull swings and 2 squats.
- Set three: perform 3 kettlebell high pull swings and 3 squats.
- Continue to 25 reps of swings and 25 squats in between the two motions.
- Other options include exchanging the swing for a KB Figure Eight.

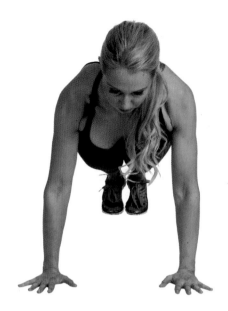

KB TGU Flow 1

Set one:
- Perform a Turkish get-up, steps 1–6, all the way up to standing.
- Before going down, press the kettlebell down to racked position.
- Then swing the kettlebell down into a single-arm kettlebell swing.
- After you finish the swing, clean the kettlebell back to racked position.
- Then press the kettlebell overhead.
- Continue Turkish get-up steps 1–6 down to the start of your TGU.

After that . . .
- The next time you get up, do 2 swings, then 3, and all the way up to 10 swings.
- This will be a total of 10 reps of the TGU on one side.
- Continue to the other side for the same number of reps.

KB TGU Flow 2

Set one:
- Perform a Turkish get-up, steps 1–6, all the way up to standing.
- Before going down, press the kettlebell down to racked position.

- Execute one lateral lunge (perform all lunges on the same side that the kettlebell is racked).
- Perform one rear lunge.
- Complete one 45-degree lunge.
- Then press the kettlebell overhead.
- Continue steps 1–6 down to the start of your TGU.

After that . . .
- The next time you get up, do 2 of each lunge, then 3, and all the way up to 6 lateral, rear, and 45-degree lunges.
- Execute a total of 6 reps of the TGU and lunges on one side.
- Continue to the other side for the same number of reps (remember to switch the side of your lunges).

KB TGU Flow 3

Set one:
- Perform a Turkish get-up, steps 1–6, all the way up to standing.
- Before going down, shift your feet 45 degrees into a windmill stance.
- Look up to the kettlebell as you execute a windmill.
- After the windmill, come back to center and do a push press.
- After you finish the swing, bring the kettlebell back overhead.
- Continue steps 1–6 down to the start of your TGU.

After that . . .
- The next time you get up, do 2 windmills and 2 push presses, then 3, and all the way up to 8 windmills and push presses.
- This will be a total of 8 reps of the TGU on one side.
- Continue to the other side for the same number of reps.

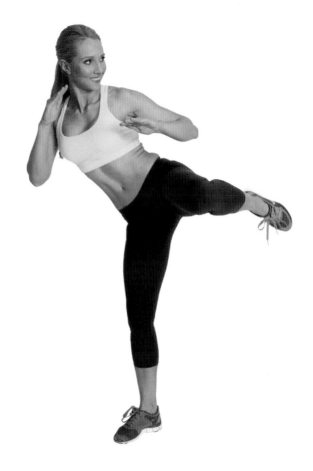

Sprawl Flow 1

- Perform 1 sprawl.
- Come up and do a squat.
- From the squat, do a vertical jump up.
- Jump back down into a squat, and from the squat, jump back into a plank.
- From the plank, do a push-up.
- From the push-up, stop and count to 15 (holding a plank).
- Bring one foot up to the knee in a spiderman push-up, then the other.
- Then push yourself back up to standing and execute 2 sprawls, followed by the same exact flow.
- Continue until you have gotten up to 20 sprawls at the top of each flow.
- Use modifications anywhere that is necessary.

Sprawl Flow 2

- Perform one sprawl.
- Come up and perform a surfer.
- Come up and alternate two snap kicks on each leg.
- Then do two crescent kicks each leg.
- Perform one more sprawl and then step back into a plank. Hold the plank for 10 seconds.
- Press your body to the ground and turn over, holding a gymnastics hollow for 10 seconds.
- Come back for your next set of the same motion as before, except this time increase your plank and hollow hold by 10 seconds, up to a 20-second hold.
- Continue all the way up to a 60-second hold for each, the plank and the hollow.
- This will be a total of 6 flows, and an increase in hold time for each.

Sprawl Flow 3

- Perform 1 sprawl.
- Come up and perform 10 alternating knees.
- After that, jump or step back into a leopard and perform 2 leopard kick-outs.
- Come back up and do 10 more alternating knees.
- Continue back down to the sprawl and repeat the full flow, except each time add 2 more leopard kicks until you reach 20 total.

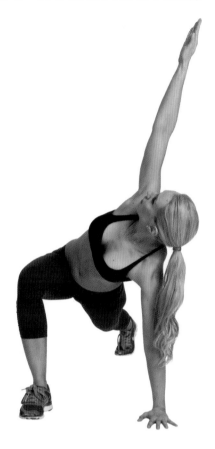

Squat Thruster Flow 1

- You will need two kettlebells.
- Perform a squat thruster.
- Follow immediately with a push press.
- Follow up with a simple press.
- Bring the kettlebells down to racked position.
- Swing them down and perform 1 full double KB swing.
- On the next swing perform a high pull.
- After the high pull clean the kettlebells up and continue on to your next rep, starting back with a squat thruster.
- This time, perform two squat thrusters.
- Keep building the squat thruster reps at the top of the motion until you execute 10 squats.

Squat Thruster Flow 2

- You will need two kettlebells.
- Perform a squat thruster.
- Follow immediately with a deep squat.
- From the squat, holding the kettlebells racked up tight to the body, perform a rear lunge to push kick on each leg.
- Follow up with a simple press from standing.
- Drop the kettlebells into a swing.
- Clean the kettlebells back up and continue to your second set of the thruster flow, but this time complete 2 thrusters.
- With every set add another thruster, until you finish at 10 total.

BURN 500 FLOW: BOTTOMS-UP RAISE/TRUE HIGH PULL FLOW

Bottoms-Up Raise/True High Pull Flow 1

- Perform a bottoms-up raise (also called the true high pull).
- At the bottom of the motion, after you have performed the first rep, catch the kettlebell up mid-racked.
- From mid-racked position perform a halo to the left and then a halo to the right.
- After the halo slide the kettlebell down to hanging and perform 3 kettlebell swings.
- Catch the kettlebell back up to mid-racked position and press it overhead.
- Slide the kettlebell back down and continue back to a bottoms-up raise.
- This time perform 2 KB bottoms-up raises, then 3, and on all the way up to 10.

Bottoms-Up Raise/True High Pull Flow 2

- Perform a bottoms-up raise (also called the true high pull).
- At the bottom of the motion, after you perform the first rep, catch the kettlebell up mid-racked.
- Continue down to a deck squat.
- Go back down in a deck squat but come up in a jiujitsu sit-up.
- Continue, but in each rep add more reps to your jiujitsu sit-up or your deck squat (all the way up to 10).

Keep in mind as you execute these flows that not all motions can be combined. Prime examples include a row and a swing; the two motions are great but cannot flow from one to the next. Instead they need to be performed one to the next, not one with the next. So if you are combining motions in a flow, stick to the preset flow patterns we have given you here.

So now that you have these, use them to BURN 500 by combining any 3 flows and getting your sweat on!

CHAPTER 11

15-MINUTE WORKOUTS THAT WORK

Your Super HIIT Workouts—No Excuses, Just Results!

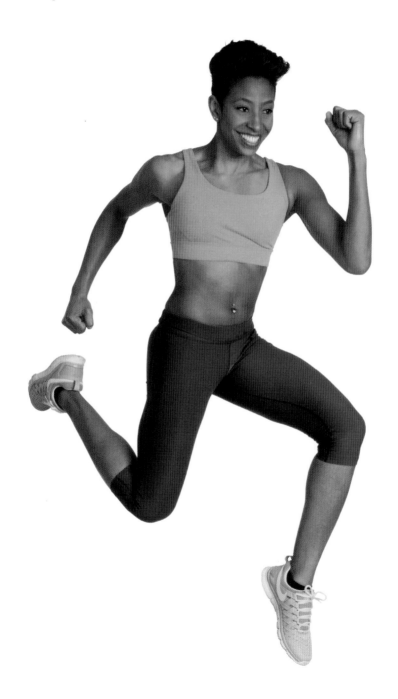

"I don't have time." "I have to wake up early." "My boss made me stay late." "I have a project." "My kids need my attention." " I'm tired." "I'm out of shape." Does that sound even a tad bit familiar? One of the greatest excuses we hear is *"I just don't have the time; I have too many other pressures right now."*

Here is my answer to that: the greater the things you do, the greater the amount of success you will see in your life. It's easy to become overwhelmed with pressure from daily responsibilities—both at work and at home. It doesn't help to look at exercise as just another burden! Just as eating, showering, and brushing your teeth are part of the daily routine of taking care of yourself, so should exercise be a priority in your life! But, just to make it a little bit easier on you, I have created an assortment of 15-minute exercises.

We believe what we want to believe; however, you are far more likely to believe something if you say it to yourself. As a simple exercise, if you say to yourself one morning, or perhaps one evening after work, any of these phrases: "I'm tired. I can't work out today. It's too early. It's too late," then you will undoubtedly feel tired and your mind will shift, making the decision that you are too busy to exercise today. If, however, you take the same exact day and say to yourself, "I feel great! It's going to be a busy day and the best thing I can do is start with an energy-pumping workout. The second I get this workout done, I will have more energy to tackle my day," then you will not only find time to work out, but you will also send a signal to your brain that will grant the body with the energy you need to complete the workout, be it in the morning before you start your day or in the evening as a stress reliever.

> Remember that exercise makes you more clear-headed and more productive! For every 15, 25, 30, or 60 minutes you spend moving and training your own body, you will get more energy to be a better and more productive mother, daughter, wife, coworker, boss, and person.

IS 15 MINUTES ENOUGH?

It is true that most everyone is hard-pressed for time. But luckily, with the use of such an efficient tool as the kettlebell, and the combination of high-intensity interval training (HIIT), not only will you have time to work out, but also the pace and motions will provide your body with the energy you need to sustain the rest of your day. With the right tools, motions, and time intervals, a 15-minute workout can turn your body into a powerhouse of strength, endurance, and lean muscle. The key, of course, is to include the right rest-to-work ratio and also to perform the correct exercises in the right succession.

So, can you burn calories, build muscle, and develop strength in 15 minutes? YES, of course you can, and you will!

To help you get the most out of your time, we'll be combining the following concepts from our trademark KB system:

- **Kettlebell Exercises:** high in intensity, ballistic, and weight training; multijoint motions.
- **Martial Arts Plyometrics:** safer, more fun, and a perfect complement to the kettlebell.
- **Variations of HIIT Time Intervals:** different ratios of work-to-rest periods call upon different energy systems and cause specific adaptations. In this book, these will be variations from track and field, sports science, and martial arts time variations.

TIME INTERVALS

Studies have shown that short yet intense workouts improve athletic capacity and conditioning, improve glucose metabolism, and improve fat burning. Different ratios of work-to-rest periods call upon different energy systems and cause specific adaptations. Many of those adaptations include building muscle and burning fat, as well as performance enhancement in many sports. This happens because structured patterns of work and rest periods elicit a desired response from the body. The work-to-rest time intervals we will use in our 15-minute workouts are specifically geared to getting the body to build a postworkout fat-burning response in the body.

Another way to describe these types of workouts is by calling them your metabolic conditioning workouts. The purpose of metabolic conditioning is to maximize the efficiency of a particular energy system to perform better in sports or develop your desired physique. One added benefit is the increase of caloric burn even after the workout is finished.

Our time intervals will mainly consist of the following principles and variations of these principles:

Traditional high-intensity interval training (**HIIT**), also called high-intensity intermittent exercise (HIIE) or **sprint interval training**, is considered an enhanced form of interval training. This type of exercise alternates periods of short, intense anaerobic exercise with less-intense recovery periods. Typically it involves a rest period that is half the time of the work period. HIIT is considered a form of cardiovascular training, but due to its intensity, it does not require a traditional hour of exercise. HIIT sessions typically last between 9 to 25 minutes—any more than that and you will lower your performance and increase your risk of injury.

> Example of a HIIT exercise: 1 minute of a sprint burst followed by 30 seconds of light jogging, walking, or fully resting.

Tabata is form of HIIT training, and we will be using it a lot in the workouts in this chapter. Tabata became very popular after a 1996 study used 20 seconds of ultra-intense exercise (at an intensity of about 170% of VO_2 max) followed by 10 seconds of rest, repeated continuously for 4 minutes (8 cycles) as a more successful way to practice cardio. The most common way to perform Tabata is by doing the following:

- 5 minutes of warm-up
- 8 intervals of 20 seconds of all-out intensity exercise followed by 10 seconds of rest
- 2 minutes of cool-down or rest before beginning another set of a different Tabata or other exercises

For your 15-minute workouts, we will combine 2 to 4 exercises. All of the exercises we combine will be ones that can work together. Make sure you can execute each one individually before moving on to the combinations given here.

Your Moves*

*Use the move listed or any of the move's variations.

Box A	Box B	Box C
Use any move from chapters 4, 7, or 8.	Use any move from chapter 6.	Use any move from chapter 5.

Straight Tabata

Spend 3–5 minutes performing a light warm-up using 3–5 warm-ups from chapter 9.

Then pick 3 exercises from the boxes: one exercise from Box A, one from Box B, and one from Box C. Place them into the following module:

- Perform the first exercise you picked for 8 rounds of 20 seconds of work and 10 seconds of rest. Total: 4 minutes of work.
- Then rest for 1 minute (more advanced) to 2 minutes (more typical).
- Perform the second exercise you picked for 8 rounds of 20 seconds of work and 10 seconds of rest. Total: 4 minutes of work.
- Then rest for 1 minute (more advanced) to 2 minutes (more typical).
- Perform the third exercise you picked for 8 rounds of 20 seconds of work and 10 seconds of rest. Total: 4 minutes of work.
- Then rest for 1 minute (more advanced) to 2 minutes (more typical).
- Stretch using 3–6 cool-down stretches from chapter 9.

An example of my favorite Tabata set is the kettlebell swing!
Just swing at a work-to-rest ratio of 20 seconds of work to 10 seconds of rest for 4 full minutes.

Tabata Two

Spend 3–5 minutes performing a light warm-up using 3 to 5 warm-ups from chapter 9.

Then pick 3 exercises from the boxes: two exercises from Box A, two from Box B, and two from Box C. Place them into the following module:

- Perform the first and second exercises you picked for 8 rounds of 20 seconds of work and 10 seconds of rest. Total: 4 minutes of work.
- Then rest for 1 minute (more advanced) to 2 minutes (more typical).
- Perform the third and fourth exercises you picked for 8 rounds of 20 seconds of work and 10 seconds of rest. Total: 4 minutes of work.
- Then rest for 1 minute (more advanced) to 2 minutes (more typical).
- Perform the fifth and sixth exercises you picked for 8 rounds of 20 seconds work and 10 seconds rest. Total: 4 minutes of work.
- Then rest for 1 minute (more advanced) to 2 minutes (more typical).
- Stretch using 3–6 cool-down stretches from chapter 9.

40/20 HIT

Spend 3–5 minutes performing a light warm-up using 3–5 warm-ups from chapter 9.

Then pick 6 exercises from the boxes: two exercises from Box A, two from Box B, and two from Box C. Place them into the following module:

Round 1
- 40 seconds of exercise #1 / 20 second rest
- 40 seconds of exercise #2 / 20 second rest
- 40 seconds of exercise #3 / 20 second rest

Round 2
- 40 seconds of exercise #4 / 20 second rest
- 40 seconds of exercise #5 / 20 second rest
- 40 seconds of exercise #6 / 20 second rest

After that . . .
- Rest for 2–3 minutes as needed.
- Repeat rounds 1 and 2 again.
- Stretch using 3–6 stretches from chapter 9.

KB 20-to-2

Spend 3–5 minutes performing a light warm-up using 3 to 5 warm-ups from chapter 9.

Pick any 2 exercises, the first from Box A and the other from Box B or Box C, and place them into the following module:

- Begin by performing 20 reps of exercise #1 and immediately follow with 20 reps of exercise #2.
- Keeping good form, continue to reduce the number of each set by 2.
- Set two would be 18 reps of exercise #1 and 18 of exercise #2.
- Continue on until you hit 0 reps.
- Our favorite combo? The kettlebell swing and the push-up (use modified when needed).
- If using a static motion like a plank, hold for 20 seconds instead.
- Stretch using 3–6 cool-down stretches from chapter 9.

Spend 3–5 minutes performing a light warm-up using 3–5 warm-ups from chapter 9.

Pick 11 exercises, 5 from Box A, 3 from Box B, and 3 from Box C, and place them into the following module:

- Perform each exercise for 1 minute straight. Use modifications whenever needed and keep an eye on form.
- Rest for 30 seconds between each exercise.
- For an advanced version, you can try to only rest for 20 seconds.
- Continue to perform all 10 exercises consecutively in the 1 minute of work with 30 seconds of rest time interval.
- Choose your exercises in the following order:

   1. Box A
   2. Box B
   3. Box A
   4. Box C
   5. Box A
   6. Box B
   7. Box A
   8. Box C
   9. Box A
   10. Box B
   11. Box C
- Stretch using 3–6 cool-down stretches from chapter 9.

KB Trademark HIIT

Circuit Style
Spend 3–5 minutes performing a light warm-up using 3–5 warm-ups from chapter 9.

Pick 4 exercises, 2 from Box A, 1 from Box B, and 1 from Box C, and place them into the following module:

- Set up a circuit where you will go from one exercise to another and perform each one for 1 minute straight.
- Once you have completed the first round (a total of 4 minutes of work), rest for 1 minute.
- Continue to repeat the circuit twice more with a minute break between the circuits.
- Stretch using 3–6 stretches from chapter 9.

Okay—so go on! Get started . . . 15 minutes from now you'll be drenched in sweat and FINISHED! Imagine how good you will feel!

CHAPTER 12

YOUR 4-WEEK PLAN

See Results in 4 Weeks with These Beginner, Intermediate, and Advanced Plans

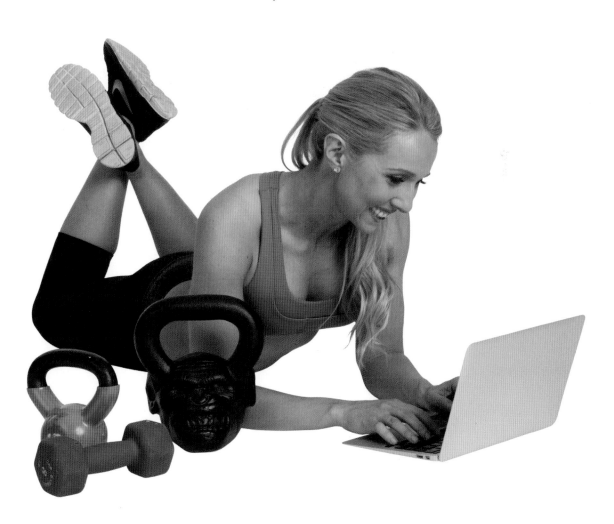

Designed to blast fat and tone muscle, the plan in this chapter is simple to follow and can be accomplished from home, at the gym, or even at the park (just don't forget to bring your trusty kettlebell with you).

We have established your exercises in the previous chapters, and have even given you some no-excuses faster workout options in chapters 10 and 11. In this chapter, we will establish a workout schedule for the next 4 weeks. There will be several options so that you can start at beginner and then graduate to intermediate and advanced time intervals and variations. You can also start at the more advanced level and then continue to the maintenance plan, which provides more options and allows you to "live" with your workouts and incorporate a routine into your life, rather than revolve your life around working out.

To help you understand which level you are, follow these guidelines:

Advanced: You fall into this category if you have your training days on lock. You work out on specific days at specific times, and your interests are also athletic. You crave and live an active lifestyle. You have no real pain or muscle/joint overuse issues (remember that even if you are highly active, you can suffer from pain or imbalances—and in that case it might be beneficial to start from the beginning).

Intermediate: You fall into this category if you work out, but not systematically. You fall in and out of exercise; sometimes you'll work out four times a week, and some weeks it may be a struggle to get to the gym once or twice. You may be active, but you don't follow a routine or work out with any real consistency.

Beginner: You fall in this category if you have not taken part in an active lifestyle in a long time, or ever. (That's okay! You're changing that now.) You have not been specifically active and are sedentary in your daily life. You don't walk much, and working out isn't habitual.

In some workouts there are modifications for beginners and options for intermediate and advanced individuals.

YOUR WORKOUTS: LET'S SWEAT!

Workout 1

For this workout, you will use a timer.

You will be working each move for 1 full minute.

Your rest will depend on your level of fitness:
- Beginner: rest for 30 seconds between each minute.
- Intermediate: rest for 15 seconds between each minute.
- Advanced: do not rest until the first full round is done.
- Rest for 45 seconds to 1 minute, as needed, between sets.

1. Standard Kettlebell Swing
2. Leopard Kick-Out
3. Bird Dog
4. Alternating Rear Lunges to Press
5. Leopard Burpee

Rest for 2 minutes and repeat 3 times for beginner and intermediate.
Repeat for 4 rounds if advanced.

Workout 2

For this workout, you will work for reps and sets and sometimes time.

Reps:
- With ballistics (all variations of swings), work for 1 minute straight, or accomplish 25–35 reps depending on kettlebell weight.
- With nonweighted motions like burpees, surfers, or leopards and others like these, work for 1 straight minute with good form.
- With all other exercises, work within an 8–15 rep range, but you should be maxing out by then!

How it works:
- Perform 2–3 sets of each if you are a beginner/intermediate.
- Perform 3–4 sets of each if you are advanced.

- Do not move on to the next exercise until all reps from the first exercise are done.
- Rest for 45 seconds to 1 minute, as needed, between sets.

1. Dead Lift
2. Row (Double KB)/Alternating Sides
3. Goblet Squat
4. Push-Up
5. Single-Leg Dead Lift (do each side separately)
6. Double KB Press

Workout 3

For this workout, you will work for reps and sets and sometimes time.

Reps:
- With ballistics (all variations of swings), work for 1 minute straight, or accomplish 25–35 reps depending on kettlebell weight.
- With nonweighted motions like burpees, surfers, or leopards and others like these, work for 1 straight minute with good form.
- With all other exercises, work within an 8–15 rep range, but you should be maxing out by then!

How it works:
- Perform 2–3 sets of each if you are a beginner/intermediate.
- Perform 3–4 sets of each if you are advanced.
- Do not move on to the next exercise until all reps from the first exercise are done.
- Rest for 45 seconds to 1 minute, as needed, between sets.

1. Kettlebell Swing (standard)
2. Walking Lunges
3. Controlled Fire Drill
4. Windmill (do each side)
5. Kettlebell Bridge
6. Kettlebell Twist

Workout 4

For this workout, you will work for reps and sets and sometimes time.

Reps:
- With ballistics (all variations of swings), work for 1 minute straight, or accomplish 25–35 reps depending on kettlebell weight.
- With nonweighted motions like burpees, surfers, or leopards and others like these, work for 1 straight minute with good form.
- With all other exercises, work within an 8–15 rep range, but you should be maxing out by then!

How it works:
- Perform 2–3 sets of each if you are a beginner/intermediate.
- Perform 3–4 sets of each if you are advanced.
- Do not move on to the next exercise until all reps from the first exercise are done.
- Rest for 45 seconds to 1 minute, as needed, between sets.

1. Bottoms-Up Raise
2. 1-Inch Butt Lifter (both sides)
3. Turkish Get-Up (both sides)
4. Killer Combo
5. Sprawl to Kick
6. Side Plank

Workout 5

For this workout, you will work for reps and sets and sometimes time.

Reps:
- With ballistics (all variations of swings), work for 1 minute straight, or accomplish 25–35 reps depending on kettlebell weight.
- With nonweighted motions like burpees, surfers, or leopards and others like these, work for 1 straight minute with good form.
- With all other exercises work within an 8–15 rep range, but you should be maxing out by then!

How it works:
- Perform 2–3 sets of each if you are a beginner/intermediate.
- Perform 3–4 sets of each if you are advanced.
- Do not move on to the next exercise until all reps from the first exercise are done.
- Rest for 45 seconds to 1 minute, as needed, between sets.

1. Hammer Chop with Halo
2. Walking Lunges
3. Surfer
4. KB Warrior
5. Cat Squat
6. Leopards

Workout 6

For this workout, you will use a timer. You will be working each move for 1 full minute.

Your rest will depend on your level of fitness:
- Beginner: rest for 30 seconds between each minute.
- Intermediate: rest for 15 seconds between each minute.
- Advanced: do not rest until the first full round is done.
- Rest for 45 seconds to 1 minute, as needed, between sets.

1. Gun Slingers
2. Spider Switches to Push-Ups
3. Plank
4. Crescent Kick to Crescent Lunge
5. High Pulls

- Rest for 2 minutes and repeat 3 times for beginners and intermediate.
- Repeat for 4 rounds if advanced.

Workout 7

For this workout, you will use a timer. You will be working each move for 1 full minute.

Your rest will depend on your level of fitness:
- Beginner: rest for 30 seconds between each minute.
- Intermediate: rest for 15 seconds between each minute.
- Advanced: do not rest until the first full round is done.
- Rest for 45 seconds to 1 minute, as needed, between sets.

1. Squat to Kick Combo
2. 30-30-30 Push-Up
3. Swing Switches
4. Lunge to Push Kick
5. Turkish Get-Up

- Rest for 2 minutes and repeat 3 times for beginners and intermediate.
- Repeat for 4 rounds if advanced.

Workout 8

For this workout, you will use a timer. You will be working each move for 1 full minute.

Your rest will depend on your level of fitness:
- Beginner: rest for 30 seconds between each minute.
- Intermediate: rest for 15 seconds between each minute.
- Advanced: do not rest until the first full round is done.
- Rest for 45 seconds to 1 minute, as needed, between sets.

1. Double KB High Pulls, or alternate through the swing switch with a single kettlebell
2. MMA Sit-Up
3. Speed Skaters
4. Double KB Clean and Press, or alternate through the swing switch with a single kettlebell
5. Sumo Squat to Sumo Jack

- Rest for 2 minutes and repeat 3 times for beginners and intermediate.
- Repeat for 4 rounds if advanced.

Workout 9

For this workout, you will use a timer. You will be working each move for 1 full minute.

Your rest will depend on your level of fitness:
- Beginner: rest for 30 seconds between each minute.
- Intermediate: rest for 15 seconds between each minute.
- Advanced: do not rest until the first full round is done.
- Rest for 45 seconds to 1 minute, as needed, between sets.

1. Suitcase Swing Left
2. Suitcase Swing Right
3. Snap Kick to Fire Drill
4. Gymnastic Hollow Hold (10 second hold/5 second rest, continuing for 1 minute)
5. Squat Thruster

- Rest for 2 minutes and repeat 3 times for beginners and intermediate.
- Repeat for 4 rounds if advanced.

Workout 10

For this workout, you will work for reps and sets.

- Perform 2–3 sets of each if you are a beginner/intermediate.
- Perform 3–4 sets of each if you are advanced.
- Do not move on to the next exercise until all reps from the first exercise are done.
- Rest for 45 seconds to 1 minute, as needed, between sets.

1. KB Catch Swing to Squat
2. Mermaid
3. Overhead Sit-Up
4. Jiujitsu Sit-Up or Deck Squat
5. Lateral Lunges (do both sides)
6. Leopard Push-Up

4-WEEK SUCCESS PLAN FOR A TOTAL-BODY TRANSFORMATION

WEEK ONE		
	Monday	Workout 1
	Tuesday	Any 15-Minute workout
	Wednesday	Workout 2
	Thursday	Workout 8
	Friday	Any Burn 500 workout
	Saturday	Workout 4
	Sunday	REST or do a recovery workout from chapter 9

WEEK TWO		
	Monday	Any Burn 500 workout
	Tuesday	Workout 5
	Wednesday	Workout 6
	Thursday	Any 15-Minute workout
	Friday	Workout 2
	Saturday	Workout 7
	Sunday	REST or do a recovery workout from chapter 9

WEEK THREE		
	Monday	Workout 3
	Tuesday	Workout 9
	Wednesday	Any Burn 500 workout
	Thursday	Workout 2
	Friday	Workout 10
	Saturday	REST or any 15-Minute workout or do a recovery workout from chapter 9
	Sunday	Any 15-Minute workout

WEEK FOUR		
	Monday	Workout 6
	Tuesday	Any 15-Minute workout
	Wednesday	Workout 4
	Thursday	Workout 8
	Friday	Workout 5
	Saturday	Any Burn 500 workout
	Sunday	REST or do a recovery workout from chapter 9

4-WEEK PROGRAM AB FOCUS

WEEK ONE	Monday	Use one ab workout from chapter 5
	Tuesday	Any 15-Minute workout
	Wednesday	Workout 2
	Thursday	Workout 8
	Friday	Any Burn 500 workout
	Saturday	Use one ab workout from chapter 5
	Sunday	REST or do a recovery workout from chapter 9

WEEK TWO	Monday	Any Burn 500 workout
	Tuesday	Use one ab workout from chapter 5
	Wednesday	Workout 6
	Thursday	Any 15-Minute workout
	Friday	Use one ab workout from chapter 5
	Saturday	Workout 7
	Sunday	REST or do a recovery workout from chapter 9

WEEK THREE	Monday	Use one ab workout from chapter 5
	Tuesday	Workout 9
	Wednesday	Any Burn 500 workout
	Thursday	Workout 2
	Friday	Use one ab workout from chapter 5
	Saturday	REST or any 15-Minute workout or do a recovery workout from chapter 9
	Sunday	Any 15-Minute workout or do a recovery workout from chapter 9

WEEK FOUR	Monday	Workout 6
	Tuesday	Any 15-Minute workout
	Wednesday	Workout 4
	Thursday	Use one ab workout from chapter 5
	Friday	Workout 5
	Saturday	Any Burn 500 workout
	Sunday	REST or do a recovery workout from chapter 9

4-WEEK PROGRAM LEG FOCUS

WEEK ONE		
	Monday	Use one leg workout from chapter 7
	Tuesday	Any 15-Minute workout
	Wednesday	Workout 2
	Thursday	Workout 8
	Friday	Any Burn 500 workout
	Saturday	Use one leg workout from chapter 7
	Sunday	REST or do a recovery workout from chapter 9

WEEK TWO		
	Monday	Any Burn 500 workout
	Tuesday	Use one leg workout from chapter 7
	Wednesday	Workout 6
	Thursday	Any 15-Minute workout
	Friday	Workout 3
	Saturday	Use one leg workout from chapter 7
	Sunday	REST or do a recovery workout from chapter 9

WEEK THREE		
	Monday	Use one leg workout from chapter 7
	Tuesday	Workout 9
	Wednesday	Any Burn 500 workout
	Thursday	Workout 1
	Friday	Use one leg workout from chapter 7
	Saturday	REST or any 15-Minute workout or do a recovery workout from chapter 9
	Sunday	Any 15-Minute workout or do a recovery workout from chapter 9

WEEK FOUR		
	Monday	Workout 6
	Tuesday	Any 15-Minute workout
	Wednesday	Workout 4
	Thursday	Use one leg workout from chapter 7
	Friday	Workout 5
	Saturday	Any Burn 500 workout
	Sunday	REST or do a recovery workout from chapter 9

4-WEEK PROGRAM ARM FOCUS

WEEK ONE	Monday	Workout 1
	Tuesday	Any 15-Minute workout
	Wednesday	Use one arm workout from chapter 6
	Thursday	Workout 8
	Friday	Any Burn 500 workout
	Saturday	Use one arm workout from chapter 6
	Sunday	REST or do a recovery workout from chapter 9

WEEK TWO	Monday	Any Burn 500 workout
	Tuesday	Use one arm workout from chapter 6
	Wednesday	Workout 6
	Thursday	Any 15-Minute workout
	Friday	Use one arm workout from chapter 6
	Saturday	Workout 7
	Sunday	REST or do a recovery workout from chapter 9

WEEK THREE	Monday	Use one arm workout from chapter 6
	Tuesday	Workout 9
	Wednesday	Any Burn 500 workout
	Thursday	Use one arm workout from chapter 6
	Friday	Workout 10
	Saturday	Any 15-Minute workout
	Sunday	REST or any 15-Minute workout or do a recovery workout from chapter 9

WEEK FOUR	Monday	Workout 6
	Tuesday	REST or do a recovery workout from chapter 9
	Wednesday	Use one arm workout from chapter 6
	Thursday	Workout 8
	Friday	Workout 5
	Saturday	Any Burn 500 workout
	Sunday	REST or do a recovery workout from chapter 9

4-WEEK PROGRAM GLUTE FOCUS

WEEK ONE	Monday	Workout 1
	Tuesday	Any 15-Minute workout
	Wednesday	Use one glute workout from chapter 8
	Thursday	Workout 8
	Friday	Any Burn 500 workout
	Saturday	Use one glute workout from chapter 8
	Sunday	REST or do a recovery workout from chapter 9

WEEK TWO	Monday	Any Burn 500 workout
	Tuesday	Use one glute workout from chapter 8
	Wednesday	Workout 6
	Thursday	Any 15-Minute workout
	Friday	Use one glute workout from chapter 8
	Saturday	Workout 7
	Sunday	REST or do a recovery workout from chapter 9

WEEK THREE	Monday	Use one glute workout from chapter 8
	Tuesday	Workout 9
	Wednesday	Any Burn 500 workout
	Thursday	Use one glute workout from chapter 8
	Friday	Workout 10
	Saturday	REST or any 15-Minute workout or do a recovery workout from chapter 9
	Sunday	Any 15-Minute workout

WEEK FOUR	Monday	Workout 6
	Tuesday	Any 15-Minute workout
	Wednesday	Use one glute workout from chapter 8
	Thursday	Workout 8
	Friday	Use one glute workout from chapter 8
	Saturday	Any Burn 500 workout
	Sunday	REST or do a recovery workout from chapter 9

AND NOW WHAT?

Okay, now that you have finished your 4-week plan, what happens next?

First of all, you have an encyclopedia of workouts to carry with you through every step of your life and your goals.

You can pull workouts and moves from each chapter and continue to stay active for the rest of your life.

In the maintenance discussion that follows, I will tell you that the best formula would be to pick any of the countless workouts you have in this book and use them to stay on track by training 3–4 times a week. You can also begin to use the moves illustrated and the information you have learned to make your own workouts.

A MAINTENANCE PLAN FOR LIFELONG SUCCESS!

Above all else, it's important to understand that you should be active and mobile every single day. Your health is a lifelong process, not something that you cultivate for 30 days and then abandon. Your body will be with you for the rest of your life, so you must take care of it for as long as you live in it!

Having said that, the maintenance workout program is attainable and sustainable. Now that you've created good exercise habits (and good nutrition, covered in the next chapter), you'll continue to make strides while training a minimum of 3–4 times a week because you'll be giving it your all with every motion and rep.

I have provided a sample maintenance workout month. Having tested this program extensively, I can honestly say that it's okay for you to do workouts on back-to-back days, and it's equally okay to take a day or more off in between sessions. You can also pick ANY workout you want to complete each day; what's listed is merely a model. Ideally, you will complete these workouts in 2 weeks, spacing them out so that you work out 3–4 times per week (and never more than once per day).

Learn to listen to your body! As you begin to love working out, your body will begin to look forward to this time. Figure out what workout you're craving, and go for it! Learn to use your workouts as a time of self-discovery.

However, keep in mind that in order to keep your results, you must adhere to your daily maintenance nutrition plan (covered in the next chapter) while consistently working out 3–4 times a week. Do NOT skip weeks of workouts. You must also stay active throughout your day.

AFTER YOUR INITIAL 4 WEEKS

Remember, you only have one body, and it's the one you have been so dedicated to for the past month. You have already made the changes, lived the program, and seen the amazing results.

Can you continue on this journey? Of course you can! You're already doing it! You couldn't have achieved what you've done without beginning to reinvent your lifestyle.

Think about it: Are you the same person you were 4 weeks ago? Does your mind feel the same? Does your body feel the same? Did you form new habits? Do you have new energy? Do you feel better? Do you look the same? Do you move the same? Do you crave the same foods?

If you've stuck with the program this far, you've already made a commitment to yourself. You have rid yourself of many poor habits and realized how much better you feel, move, live, sleep, and function. That commitment and change is a part of you now.

From here on out, your goal is to continue on this journey—think process, not product. Once you reach a goal, make another. No pressure, just fun. From here on out, your life should be full of motion, discovery, and fitness. Enjoy your body! Enjoy your lifestyle! Take advantage of your energy!

In this final maintenance phase, you will continue to challenge yourself; if you started at beginner, try the intermediate and advanced workouts, and focus on your breath, form, and intensity. You have to continue to discover yourself, as you did when we first started the program. Simply follow the maintenance calendars and general guidelines listed here.

4-WEEK SAMPLE MAINTENANCE PLAN

WEEK ONE		
	Monday	Workout 1 or 2
	Tuesday	Any 15-Minute workout
	Wednesday	Workout 7
	Thursday	REST or do any 15-Minute workout
	Friday	Any Burn 500 workout
	Saturday	Workout 4, or if you're in a hurry any 15-Minute workout
	Sunday	REST or do a recovery workout from chapter 9

WEEK TWO		
	Monday	Any Burn 500 workout
	Tuesday	Any Burn 500 workout
	Wednesday	Workout 6
	Thursday	Any 15-Minute workout
	Friday	Workout 4
	Saturday	Workout 10
	Sunday	REST or do a recovery workout from chapter 9

WEEK THREE		
	Monday	Any 15-Minute workout
	Tuesday	Workout 9
	Wednesday	Any Burn 500 workout
	Thursday	Any 15-Minute workout
	Friday	REST or any Burn 500 workout
	Saturday	REST or any 15-Minute workout or do a recovery workout from chapter 9
	Sunday	REST or any 15-Minute workout or do a recovery workout from chapter 9

WEEK FOUR		
	Monday	Workout 6
	Tuesday	REST
	Wednesday	Workout 5
	Thursday	Workout 3
	Friday	Any 15-Minute workout
	Saturday	Any Burn 500 workout
	Sunday	REST or do a recovery workout from chapter 9

KETTLEBELL KICKBOXING

This calendar is just a sample; you can supplement with any workout you would like! Just make sure you get at least 2 longer workouts in a week.

DAY-TO-DAY

- Follow your clean-eating nutrition from chapter 13.
- Make time! If you're in a hurry, use chapters 9 and 10 to get your workout in.
- Work out! Follow the training program 3–4 days a week.
- Stay active throughout your day and week.
- Days off should be spent hiking, walking, and doing fun activities with family and friends!

WHEN YOU TRAVEL

You have two options on trips: you can take the week off and relax, or you can take the workouts with you and train in your hotel room (or at the beach or hotel gym). If you choose to stay with your program:

- Continue to make good nutrition choices. Enjoy your food, but keep your indulgences to a minimum.
- If you're traveling for work, continue your workouts in your hotel and maintain a healthy diet.
- If you're traveling for two or more weeks, try to squeeze in workouts and stay on top of your nutrition.

TRAVEL WORKOUT PLAN

Here are two no-excuses travel workouts you can perform without any equipment.

For these workouts, you will work for reps and sets.

- Perform 2–3 sets of each if you are a beginner.
- Perform 3–4 sets of each if you are advanced.
- Do not move on to the next exercise until all reps from the first exercise are done.
- Rest for 45 seconds to 1 minute, as needed between sets.

Travel Workout 1

1. Push-Ups: modified or regular
2. Sumo Squat to Sumo Jack
3. Leopard Push-Up
4. Rear Lunges to Push Kicks
5. Snap Kick Thruster
6. Plank (any variation)

Travel Workout 2

1. Lateral Lunge
2. Walking Lunges
3. Surfer
4. Nonweighted KB Warrior
5. Jinga Lunges
6. Burpee with a Snap Kick

YOU MUST MOVE OUTSIDE OF THE GYM!

Working out systematically on a solid program like the one provided for you in this book is the key to unlocking your body's full potential. You must be on a program, and you must be committed to it, in order to achieve incredible results.

But, you cannot sit 12 hours a day (e.g., spend it all sleeping, watching TV, working at a desk, eating lunch in a chair) and then work out/move 1 hour a day and expect to make lasting changes in your life.

MOVE! **Movement is life!**

Your Kettlebell Kickboxing workouts will help you look, feel, and move better, with no pain. Move faster. Be active. Be mobile. Be fit and feel strong. To get there, you must also make it a point to move throughout your day—on your days off especially. Be a great example to your family and friends and aim to live an active lifestyle. This will help you enjoy more things as well as maintain all of that hard-earned progress you worked for in your 4-week plan and in your KB workouts.

How to stay active on your days off from working out:

- Walk to work once a week.

- Stand on the train.

- NEVER take the elevator (okay, so if you work on the 30th floor, walk up 6–10 staircases and then catch the elevator).

- Walk/play with your dog.

- Walk/play with your child.

- Go out to get lunch.

- Have an auto alert every 45 minutes on your computer or phone to GET UP and walk around office, do 50 squats, and then get back to your desk, or run in place for 2 minutes every 45 minutes.

- On Sunday, make active plans—walk to brunch or lunch, hike, bike, or play golf or baseball.

- On Saturday nights, instead of sitting at the movies, go bowling, play pool, or go dancing.

- For every drink you consume at the bar, dance five songs.

- Get RID of your couch or other unnecessary sitting-enabling furniture in the living room so you can do movement on the ground when watching TV.

- For 1 hour a day, sit on a yoga ball.

- Play-wrestle with your spouse or significant other.

- Ride a bike to pick up your groceries or do your to-do list.

- Get an outdoor hobby (there are plenty to pick from).

- Jump up and down like a kid 50 times a day.

- Skip down five blocks on your way to get your coffee in the morning.

- Carry your groceries home.

- Walk your neighbor's dog(s).

- MOVE!!!

I hope you can really incorporate this into your days and weeks. Make fit and active plans on your days off, like skiing, hiking, walking, swimming, and exploring.

CHAPTER 13

AN EXERCISE IN KETTLEBELL NUTRITION

Maximize Your Results with This KB-Approved Diet Plan

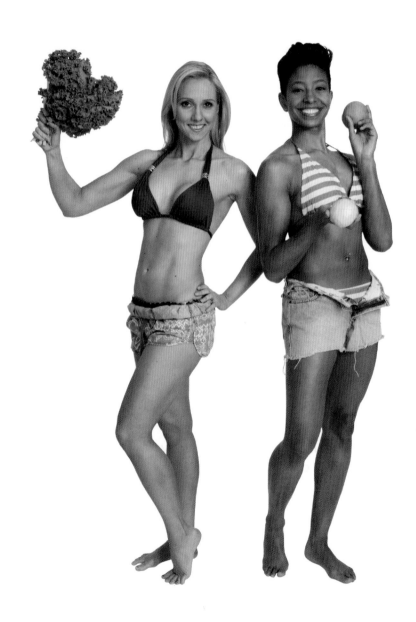

All of my Kettlebell Kickboxing home workout programs are complete with a nutrition program. The program is actually simple and details the concepts I discuss here. The only more extensive program I provide is in my 7-Day Lean DVD and nutrition program that has specific event prep and workout cleanse options. But the rest of the Kettlebell Kickboxing nutrition concepts are right here. They really are simple. They work the best with the workouts, and without using these concepts, you will not get the results you would if you successfully combined your fitness and nutrition.

Now, believe it or not, this is all you need to succeed and understand how to "eat clean" for any version of your life—whether you're a vegetarian, vegan, chocolate lover, or wine fanatic. You can have what you love and want and still be healthy and see results. Read on and you will begin to understand how simple nutrition really is.

Combine these concepts with the program and you will be shocked at how incredible your results will be and how great you will feel!

First and Foremost, Have a Fitness Mind-Set in Diet

Before we even get into any nutritional advice or guidelines, I want to discredit some of the notions that people have about diet and exercise.

Exercise decreases hunger. It should NOT inflict hunger or serve as a reason for you to eat more. So get that mentality out of your head!

- Exercise decreases hunger because it spurs the production of stimulating hormones like thyroxine, norepinephrine, and testosterone. Working out also increases your levels of the stimulating neurotransmitter dopamine. These body chemicals kill hunger even more effectively than eating does!

- Hunger often results from stress and boredom. Luckily, exercise increases serotonin levels, which helps you relax.

- Lastly, exercise should make you more aware of what you put into your body, which actually craves good food.

- Fitness, health, and wellness will never come out of starvation or deprivation diets.

MY PHILOSOPHY ON FOOD

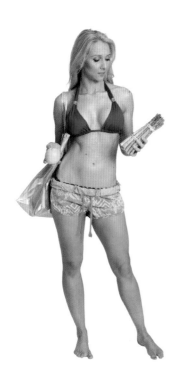

Food is a big part of our lives. I love that. You've got to be excited by the important, basic things in life, like food. The key to living well, though, is to learn to be excited by the kind of food you should be eating: good, natural, whole, real foods, not processed garbage that harms your body.

What's more, you shouldn't feel bound by either a specific food or diet. It's easy to let almost anything control and overrun your life. Many people allow food to become a dependency, a crutch, and a point of weakness. Don't let it. Approach your daily nutrition with discipline and mental fortitude. How? Through a natural and organic approach of strength and balance—the same way you set boundaries in other aspects of your life, like relationships, work, and parenting. Treat food like everything else:

- Quality over quantity
- Pleasure over pain
- Balance over stress
- Moderation over access

For many of us, this is tough. Why? Because we have spent too much time creating stress around the very thing that serves us and our bodies. Often, it's a case of too much information. We get so confused about "which diet," "which program," "what timing," "what quantity," "what quality," and "how much" that we don't stick to one thing. Instead, we constantly switch and combine things until we go numb with confusion and stress, all while seeing limited results. So, I ask you here and now to STOP! Stop letting piecemeal and random health information into your life.

Health, which includes fitness and nutrition, is a straight line. As you read about the simplicity of the nutrition guidelines, think of it as a straight line to your success. So, picture the line. Right now. Go on. Good! Now, let's visualize you at the end of that line, just like we did before. Remember how you saw yourself 7 days from now and then another 3 weeks after that? Follow the nutrition program provided here, and, along with the training and workouts from this book, it will give you everything you need for your success.

Stick with me on this, and I will help you achieve real, lasting results. Don't let anything or anyone interfere with your success!

OUR GOAL

Most people associate diets with trauma because they always seem to focus on what you *can't* eat, where you *can't* go, what you *can't* do. That shouldn't be the case. Let's take out the negatives. Your "diet" should be a lifestyle you enjoy. It should be what you *can* eat, what you *can* experience, and what you *can* try and enjoy. You should look forward to the taste of your food as well as how good food makes you feel mentally and physically. Unfortunately, many people develop close, intimate food relationships that are mentally consuming, physically exhausting, and totally unnatural. They eat (and overeat) foods that are harmful on hormonal, caloric, and glycemic levels. Often, these foods offer nothing nutritionally, and they rob people of time, health, and energy. To put it simply: these people are not in a good relationship. They have addictions to dieting, overeating, and consuming things that they know are harmful.

The key is to identify your food issues and reeducate yourself in order to form a healthy and balanced relationship with what you eat. Food presents you with an opportunity to get in touch with yourself, your health, and your body. In many cultures, food serves as a healing tool. Food brings family together, and it's often the center of celebration and new experiences. Healthy, good food can still do all of the exact same things.

Together we will identify what kind of food serves you and your body, and what kind of food can hurt you. Once you educate yourself and begin eating smart, every part of your life will change: your energy levels, your brain power, your looks, your physical strength, and even your personal relationships.

Anybody Can Eat Smart.

- First, you have to be conscious of what you're eating.
- Second, you have to understand the difference between hunger and cravings.
- Third, you have to treat food the same way you treat any other commodity in your life by not allowing it to have power over you.
- Finally, you have to ask yourself: Is this food serving me or not? Then decide if you are going to order, buy, or consume it.

Put Food in Its Place!

- Food can be social and celebratory, but it cannot be a crutch.
- Food cannot be your escape. Almost all self-destructive eating is unconscious eating, which serves no purpose and provides no pleasure. This cannot happen anymore.

CALORIES: ENERGY IN VS. ENERGY OUT

In order to get to and stay at your body's healthy weight, we need to understand a thing or two about caloric intake.

To burn off 1 pound of body fat, you need to burn about 3,500 calories. However, don't get into the misguided habit of thinking to yourself, "I'll eat this and then burn it off by doing this." This program is not designed like that, and your thought process about food and exercise shouldn't operate that way either. You cannot borrow from Paul to pay Peter, just like you cannot eat a food and then work out to burn off that food. This mentality will leave you injured, overtrained, and stressed. Furthermore, the bad foods you eat will still affect you hormonally, which means they will negatively affect how your body heals, uses and processes energy, and stores fat.

How Much Should You Eat?

What matters most in weight loss and weight management is how many calories you ingest versus how many calories you burn (**Calories In vs. Calories Out**). For our purposes, we will use the terminology: **Energy In vs. Energy Out**.

Let's Do the Math

Active people: You fall in this category if you have your training days on lock. You work out on specific days at specific times, and your interests are also athletic. You crave and live an active lifestyle. If this describes your level of activity, take your current weight and multiply it by 15.
Example: 150 pounds x 15 = 2,250 calories per day. That's the number of calories you can eat every day without gaining weight.

Moderately active people: You fall in this category if you work out, but not systematically. You fall in and out of exercise; sometimes you'll work out 4 times a week and others it may be a struggle to get to the gym once or twice. You may be active, but you don't follow a routine or work out with any real consistency. If this describes your level of activity, take your current weight and multiply it by 13.
Example: 150 pounds x 13 = 1,950 calories per day. That's the number of calories you can eat every day without gaining weight.

Inactive people: You fall in this category if you have not taken part in an active lifestyle in a long time, or ever. (That's okay! You're changing that now.) You have not been specifically active and are sedentary in your daily life. You don't walk much, and working out isn't habitual. If this describes your level of activity, take your current weight and multiply it by 11.

Example: 150 pounds x 11 = 1,650 calories per day. That's the number of calories you can eat every day without gaining weight.

The figures above are for those people looking to maintain their weight. However, let's say we are looking to lose weight. Remember: 1 pound = 3,500 calories.

In order to lose weight safely, you can cut out 400–500 calories a day through your nutrition (Energy In). You should start by getting rid of your diet's least-nutritious foods (which we're about to cover). You can then subtract an additional 500–1,000 calories a day by working out (Energy Out). You can expend these calories through your KB workouts, which metabolically add muscle and shed fat simultaneously. This is the safe and healthy way to lose weight. What's more, by cutting out foods that aren't nutritious while training on a structured workout program, your body will build beautiful, lean muscles.

During this process, it's essential that you do not overtrain or undereat. If you begin to use these numbers to starve yourself or overtrain, it will become harder for you to lose weight in the future. It will also be more difficult to maintain a healthy weight down the road. Patience is key! Controlled methods lead to lasting results you can adjust to and live with; this is called **healthy habit**. So please, follow your training chart and make sure not to overdo the exercise portion of this process.

PUTTING IT INTO PRACTICE

Making solid and tasty nutrition choices is the first step to results.

- I'd like you to write down a list of foods and drinks you like. Go on—start writing them down.
- Once you finish, read back over your list. How many of those choices are whole, real foods (not packaged or processed)? These foods should include lean meat (like chicken and fish), eggs, dairy, vegetables, fruits, and whole grains. The drinks should include water, tea, almond milk, and naturally flavored water. Place those real foods and drinks on a separate list.
- Now, create a menu for a typical weekday using items from your "real foods" list. Think of this as the base-eating plan for the rest of your life. Don't worry—you can still have indulgent meals on a fun weekend,

birthday, date, or holiday. However, you cannot make those days and those meals the base of your food pyramid. They have to be the tip; pizza and ice cream can be the once-in-a-while meals, not the majority of your lunches and dinners. It's suddenly a lot simpler, right? Now you know that you can eat well and actually enjoy your food!

- Use the grocery list you've just made for yourself as a starting point, and make sure that 80 percent of all of your food comes from the produce aisle. Later in this book, we detail grocery lists for you, and our guidelines will help you make the right choices when you want to add your own flavors and tastes.

- Although it may seem challenging now, after following this KB cleanse, you will feel like a new person: one who isn't craving sugars and white bread on a daily basis. Believe it or not, 7 days is more than enough time to reset your cravings. As a result, your new grocery list and nutrition guidelines for the results part of this program will become far easier to sustain. What's more, the 30-day results program will allow you to reintroduce certain indulgences, like wine and sweets, back into your life, but in a way that does not allow for daily dependency.

LET'S CUT THE EMPTY CALORIES!

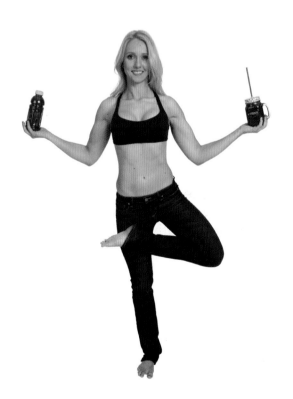

Liquids

You can kick nearly 400 calories per day just by reconsidering what you drink. The list includes juices, soda, alcoholic cocktails, and sugary coffee drinks, but it also includes sports drinks, "healthy" smoothies, and fresh juices. Even nutritious beverages can jack up your calorie count and make you pack on extra pounds. Sixteen ounces of pressed vegetable and fruit juices can add up to 440 calories. And 16 ounces of coconut water can measure in at nearly 90 calories. Most juices and flavored drinks are 200–400 calories a bottle! Does this mean you shouldn't drink healthy fruit smoothies or all-natural, organic vegetable juices? Of course not! However, the biggest mistake most people make is drinking these beverages as a snack or as part of their lunch and dinner. The truth is that a fruit and vegetable smoothie or juice should be considered a meal. Yes—the next time you drink a healthy juice, treat that as your breakfast or lunch. The general rule for an all-natural juice is that it should contain 80 percent vegetables and 20 percent fruits. If it truly is all-natural and fresh, the drink should have an expiration date of 2–3 days from the date of purchase.

Sports drinks: Unless you are a professional athlete or are participating in an outdoor activity that will last you over 60 minutes, kick the sports drinks! The calories and sugars outweigh the so-called benefits. Think of it this way: sports drinks are made for special events, like marathons. Instead, keep it simple and drink water.

Alcohol: Mixed drinks can have as many as 300 calories per serving, depending on what type of beverage you prefer. The best way to cut calories during a night out is to add ice and soda water to your mixed drink instead of juice, soda, or tonic. You can also opt for wine or ultralight beer. For a healthier twist on the mojito and other great low-calorie drink recipes, visit our blog on the Kettlebell Kickboxing website.

Milk: It does a body good, yes, but the calories add up quickly when you add milk to cereals and coffee. Even skim milk contains many calories and is high in both sugars and carbohydrates. When cutting your calories, allow yourself one glass of milk a day and be sure to account for it in your calorie allotment. For a low-sugar alternative, try all-natural, unsweetened almond milk!

Sugar

Cutting sugar alone can rid your daily diet of an extra 300–800 calories! It doesn't mean you can't ever enjoy cheesecake or your favorite cupcake. I'm not talking about the occasional indulgence; it's your daily sugar intake that matters most. Oddly enough, you probably don't even notice or particularly enjoy the daily sugar you eat as much as that apple pie you look forward to on Thanksgiving.

Did you know that food manufacturers commonly place sugars in foods you wouldn't typically label "sweets," like pita bread, soy sauce, and salad dressing? This is a good reason to read food labels. Try to avoid anything with more than 8 grams of sugar, unless it's an all-natural pressed vegetable juice, which contains natural sugars you can have daily.

The worst part? Sugar is addictive. You know that daily 3 p.m. candy or mochaccino urge? It's so hard to fight because it's not just a craving—it's an addiction! Studies have shown that sugar stimulates the same receptors and pathways activated by drugs like heroin and morphine. By constantly eating sugar, you also force your pancreas to work overtime. As you eat more sugar, it pumps out massive amounts of insulin, and eventually your body may become less sensitive to sugar.

Now, not all sugar is created equal. Natural fructose, which can be found in fruits, doesn't trigger more cravings, and fruits are full of fiber and nutrients. Fruit sugars are fine, so long as they come from real fruit. When you follow the KB program, we will ask you to maintain a balanced intake of fruit and to try to eat it during the earlier hours of the day, but the moral here is that fruit is good for you!

Sodium

Aim to keep your sodium intake under 2,500 milligrams a day. Too much salt can make you retain several pounds of extra water weight, and it can also harden your arteries. The main sodium you want to avoid is the stuff found in frozen dinners, takeout, and fast-foods. Also, be careful not to oversalt your food, and use sea salt whenever possible.

If you stick to the rule of shopping 80 percent in the produce aisle and 20 percent elsewhere, your sodium intake shouldn't be an issue. Check labels on foods, and try to avoid buying any products that have more than 300 milligrams of sodium.

Fat

Fat typically gets a bad rap because it's high in calories. However, don't fear fat. Eat foods rich in monounsaturated fats, such as olives, nuts, and avocados. With that said, portion control is key, since even the good fats are still high in calories.

Beware of hydrogenated fats! They're hidden in everything from microwave popcorn and crackers to salad dressings. Try to avoid any foods that include the terms "hydrogenated" or "partially hydrogenated" on their nutrition labels.

Here are guidelines to keep in mind when looking at the fat content listed on nutrition labels:
- Saturated fat: 0 to 0.5 grams. Aim to avoid these, if possible. They're terrible for you.
- Trans fat: absolutely 0 grams. Aim to avoid these completely.
- Polyunsaturated fat: up to 5 grams is acceptable.
- Monounsaturated fat: up to 5 grams is acceptable.
- Cholesterol: up to 20 grams is acceptable.

Proteins

Proteins are known as the building blocks of life. Once in your body, they break down into amino acids to promote cell growth and repair. Because proteins take longer to digest than carbohydrates do, they leave you feeling fuller for a longer amount of time and on fewer calories.

Whether you are a vegan, vegetarian, or omnivore, protein should be a daily component of your nutrition. Great protein sources include lean meat, chicken, fish, dairy, soy, legumes (beans), and nuts.

Be aware that some of those sources can be high in saturated fat and cholesterol. To avoid this:
- Make sure you control the portions of your dairy protein sources. Keep them to a minimum of one meal per day (or less).
- Make sure your fleshy proteins (fish, chicken, and meat) are lean cuts.
- Do not avoid protein options like quinoa and beans, which are great low-fat and high-fiber options.

Carbohydrates

Carbohydrates (starches and sugars) are fattening, mostly because they spike blood sugar levels. These periods of excessive insulin production lead to hunger cravings, overeating, and the storage of calories as body fat.

General Carbohydrate Guidelines:
- Unless it's a special dinner or day, do not mix heavy proteins (like meat) with starchy carbohydrates.
- Balance your diet by eating 70 percent nonstarchy carbs and 30 percent starchy carbs.

Non-Starchy Carbs
Although all vegetables contain starch, the following contain it in relatively small proportions:

- Asparagus*
- Beets
- Brussels sprouts
- Cabbage
- Carrots
- Kohlrabi
- Lettuce
- Okra
- Onions*
- Parsnips

- Celery*
- Chard*
- Cucumbers
- Dandelion greens
- Eggplant*
- Endive
- Jicama
- Spinach*
- String beans
- Summer squash
- Tomatoes
- Turnips
- Zucchini*
- All greens

You can eat as much of the asterisked foods (in their RAW form) as you like!

Starchy Carbs
- All foods with barley, corn, oats, rice, rye, and wheat
- Also: bananas, beans (and dried beans), chestnuts, legumes, peas, peanuts, potatoes, pumpkins, sweet potatoes, tapioca, and winter squashes

While these starchy carbs are okay, avoid the processed stuff like white bread, rice, and pasta. Instead, stick to the whole grain options.

DIETARY FIBER

The more, the better. Fiber wards off heart disease, lowers cholesterol, and controls blood sugar (which directly relates to weight management). Fiber is found in everything from fruits to beans. Here's a list of my favorite high-fiber foods:
- All-natural juices
- Whole grains (real, not refined): barley, bran, oatmeal
- Legumes: black peas, lentils, lima beans, split peas
- Vegetables: artichokes, broccoli, Brussels sprouts, peas
- Fruits: avocados, berries, pears
- Flaxseed
- Chia seeds

PUTTING ALL OF THIS TOGETHER

In the body, food has to be processed. Foods also have hormonal effects on the body. This must be taken into account when you are trying to get the best response from your digestion and your hormones. Eating whole foods helps trigger a metabolically positive response. But, in addition to that, food pairing

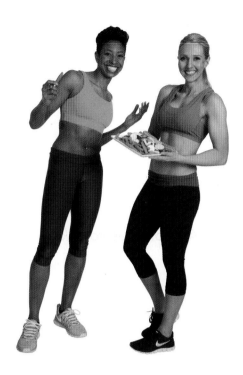

is almost equally as important. Consider your approach to foods like a chemistry project—pairing certain ones will create better responses and better digestion then pairing others. For ultimate success, aim for the following rules:

- Proteins are best eaten with vegetables or fruits. Try not to pair your proteins with starches and dairy.

- Dairy is fine, but best with berries and fruits or vegetables.

- Starches are best with veggies. If you want to enjoy bread, try to have it with vegetable soup or a hearty salad, not with meat or dairy.

THE MORAL OF THE STORY

Always look at a food's caloric content and be aware of your portions. The quality of your food is as important as its calorie count. For example, it is far more beneficial to eat a 200-calorie avocado then a 200-calorie packaged, processed imitation meal.

Calorie Breakdown
Protein: 4 calories per gram
Carbohydrates: 4 calories per gram
Fat: 9 calories per gram
Sugar: 7 calories per gram

Make good choices:
- Eat whole, natural, real food.

- Watch your portions.

- Pair foods correctly.

- Lean proteins and greens should account for 75 percent of your food choices.

- Save the sugars and high-calorie fatty foods for special occasions.

BEFORE HEADING TO THE GROCERY STORE . . .

Let's evaluate the modern grocery store. It seems to me that food manufacturers love to conceal the junk they add to processed foods. They think you're too careless to notice. Not anymore!

The Top Hidden Dangers in Store-Bought Foods

1. Sugar: Sugar is hiding in many different foods. Manufacturers understand the addictive qualities of sugar, which they use to hook you on their products. For example, sugar is hidden in salad dressings, condiments (like barbecue sauce and ketchup), and even breads like hot dog buns, pita bread, and crackers. Your only weapon as a consumer is to read your labels! Watch out for anything that sounds or looks like sucrose, fructose, maltose, lactose, and dextrose, which are hidden sugars. Also, be sure to check out a product's calorie count; if it's high in calories and you're unsure why, sugar could be the cause. Aim to eat whole grains, and get your sugar fix from natural fruits, cinnamon, and all-natural cocoa powder.

> **SCARY FACT:** The average person eats 20 teaspoons of sugar per day. Almost all of it is hidden in processed foods. That's about 70 pounds of sugar per year—enough to add (or subtract) about 40 pounds of body fat.

2. Hydrogenated Fats: Other common names for these fats are "hydrogenated oils" or "partially hydrogenated oils." Avoid foods that contain these fats listed on their nutrition labels! Hydrogenated fats are hidden in foods like chips, french fries, crackers, and fried foods.

3. Refined Grains: While it's easy to tell someone to avoid white flour, manufacturers hide processed flour in so-called whole wheat, whole grain, and multigrain foods! To be sure of what you're eating, you have to examine labels. Terms like "enriched flour," "wheat flour," and "unbleached wheat flour" all mean white flour. Sounding healthy and being healthy are two very different things!

4. Processed Foods: You can cut about 325 empty calories from your daily diet by eliminating processed foods like soda, baked goods, fruit drinks, frozen pizzas, fast-food, takeout, and flavored yogurt. Only 20 percent of your daily diet should come out of a package. That 20 percent can include different cereals as well as frozen, microwavable, and canned foods. The best of these options are vegetable steamers and healthy cereals, like unsweetened wheat puffs.

The Moral

Confused about food shopping? Don't be—your food should mainly come from the produce aisle and include vegetables, fruits, meats, chicken, fish, and eggs. Whole foods (like spinach, bananas, and apples) aren't hiding anything! Only 20 percent of your food should come in boxes or bags. Identify and avoid processed foods that contain refined grains, artificial food dyes, sweeteners (saccharin, aspartame, or sucralose) and ingredients you wouldn't cook with at home. Also, refrain from buying any packaged foods that are labeled "low-fat," "fat-free," or "preflavored." And, of course, stay away from imitation and fast foods!

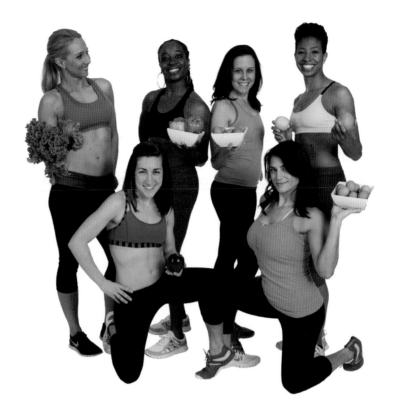

It is entirely possible to go out and eat healthy! Just keep the following information and rules in mind:

Salads

Unfortunately, the modern salad has become a high-calorie food trap. Just because something has a hint of greens and is called a salad doesn't mean it's not hiding an excess of 300–400 calories.

Many of these calories hide in the salad toppings. For example, a half cup of dried fruits typically adds 166 calories. So try to avoid the following salad components: croutons, an overabundance of nuts, deli meats, cheeses, and dried fruits.

Salad dressings can pile on an additional 150–300 calories! Instead of the usual dressings, request oil and vinegar (not vinaigrette), oil and lemon, honey mustard and lemon, or nonfat Greek yogurt (which you can season with salt and pepper). And be sure to request these dressings on the side!

Appetizers and Main Courses

It's okay to go out to restaurants! Although you should be eating clean 90 percent of time, feel free to try the more indulgent dishes during the 10 percent of the time you're allowed to treat yourself.

Dining Out: General Guidelines

- Pick restaurants that have a variety of all-natural and organic dishes.
- Order seasonal and local foods, especially when traveling. You'll get the most nutrients possible that way.
- Drink a glass of water before you order. We often mistake dehydration for hunger.
- Ask the waiter not to bring any bread.
- Share appetizers.
- Stick to one theme throughout the meal: starches and vegetables or lean proteins and vegetables.
- Don't be afraid to order an appetizer and a salad as a main course, especially since restaurant portions are typically large.
- Request dressings and sauces on the side, especially for protein-based dishes.
- Choose vegetable and protein dishes over starches, especially at dinner. You can also replace any starches with greens.
- If you're having pasta, make sure it's not mixed with proteins like meats.
- Still hungry? Get a side salad or vegetables.
- Generally, avoid dessert. If you must have something sweet, ask for a fruit plate or flavored tea.
- If you need to eat out regularly, have a go-to restaurant where the staff knows you and will make healthy food substitutions. Try to also have a go-to meal, like grilled salmon and salad.
- If you have to drink with clients regularly, get to know and love your red wines. Drink no more than 1–2 glasses in a sitting, if possible.
- Enjoy your dinner, lunch, or brunch out! But the next day, aim to cook your food and keep it simple and super healthy.

On occasion, we're all allowed to eat our favorite meals. However, "on occasion" does not mean once a day or once a week. "On occasion" means that you don't routinely preplan bad habits. It means that so long as you eat clean and lean 90 percent of the time, you can eat fast food as part of the other 10 percent.

PUTTING IT ALL TOGETHER: A FOOD LOG

Right about now, you're probably feeling overwhelmed by everything you've just read and learned. To help you simplify and combine this information, I want you to keep a food log for a week. For 7 days, I want you to write down everything you eat and drink. Additionally, I'd like you to keep track of your moods, what's stressing out, how hungry you feel before eating, and how full you feel after meals. Try to pinpoint your energy levels before and after you eat, too.

After the 7 days are up, your first step is to go through your food log with two highlighters. Use a yellow highlighter to emphasize everything you are doing "wrong" and an orange highlighter to mark everything you are doing "right," according to the KB clean-eating rules listed earlier in this chapter. Step two is simple: now that you've identified your eating habits, you can easily start making changes and breaking down walls. For every subsequent week, change one yellow portion of your log to an orange section. Sounds simple enough, no?

Example:
Week 1: In your log, you identified that your typical dinner consists of rice, beans, and meat. After evaluating your first week log, you plan to alter your eating so that Tuesday's dinner consists of meat and a large salad with homemade dressing, while Thursday's dinner consists of meat with rice and vegetables.

Week 2: In your log, you also identified a trend of 3 p.m. frappuccinos. This week, you've replaced the sugary coffee drink with a black iced coffee. You're also taking the $2.00 you save each day and putting the money toward a new pair of designer jeans.

So, that is it! And yes, if it feels simple, it's because it is. It's as simple as these guidelines. Eat clean, real, whole, natural foods. Avoid as many labels as you can, and when you see a food label—READ IT—and then ask yourself how many ingredients you actually know, understand, or use in your own cooking. If there is an overwhelming amount of ingredients with long names and unfamiliar scientific terms, you should probably not have those as a daily part of your diet.

Remember that a diet is a term for daily nutrition, not starvation and deprivation. You have to enjoy things—eat cake at a birthday party or celebrate a beautiful night out with cheese and wine. When you visit your grandparents and they serve their famous lasagna, enjoy it! Your success is reliant on your day-to-day habits, not your occasional food indulgences. Just don't make these treats a habit, and learn how to make good choices you enjoy every single day. Connect that with your workouts by setting your mind on a clear path to health and wellness and see how quickly your body becomes limitless and self-sustaining.

And *enjoy!*

CONCLUSION

*When you think you can't go any further,
or do any more—just stop thinking. You can!*

I didn't set up to write this book to just say, hey—I'm an author, I'm a writer, I'm a "fitness expert," I have a book. I set out to write this book because over the course of offering my classes, writing my weekly newsletters, and adding to our KB blog, I began to get emails and visits from women all around the world who in their own stories and journeys told me that something clicked in them, be it in the workouts at my studio, our home programs and DVDs, or the discussions I post on social media. Something clicked and they made the changes, did the workouts, followed the plan, and saw real results.

Take the journey. I do not want you to be confused by any part of this book. As I said earlier, there is too much self-serving information out there, especially when it comes to health, wellness, fitness, and nutrition. **I provide a lot of information in the book because I want you to be smart and educated about your goals, your workouts, your diet, and your body.** If you feel at all confused by anything, be assured that it is simply because you are so invested in your goals that you want to understand every single piece of the process—but that will only happen once you set out on the journey. And journeys, of course, are different from person to person. I can tell you all about my trip to Asia, or how it feels to ride an elephant. You can tell me what it's like to ski or surf or climb Everest or whatever it is you love to do; however, until we do this ourselves, the experiences we share with one another will simply be references or good stories. You read the book, you looked at the workouts, and now I urge you to take the journey.

It will not always be easy. There will be days when you'll feel exhausted or unmotivated, and other days when you will be emotional or perhaps even hopeless. The goal for us is to make sure that when you do feel this way, you use your body—exercise, movement—to get out of a rut or a bad mood. I can promise you that no matter how you feel at a given moment, the moment right after you finish your workout you will feel significantly better. You will become more motivated, creative, inspired, hopeful, and energized. Believe me.

I urge you to consider your goals, not just physical ones but also mental and spiritual ones. Find your strength, your will, your calm. Find yourself through the most natural and organic thing there is—human movement. Aim to develop yourself, and then you will undoubtedly reach every goal you set. Go into this process with an open mind and an open heart. You should know that from one great habit can stem many others. You should also know that exercise and a healthy mind-set will open up new pathways in your life.

What you expect from yourself matters. Believe it or not, you can have the strongest will and the best intentions, but if you demand the wrong thing from yourself, you can derail your goals. What I truly hope for myself, and what I fight to remember every day when I look in the mirror, is the *real* reason I work out. It's true: we all want to look great. **But,** I stand very firm on the following idea:

What I Fight to Remember Every Day

It's what your body helps you do outside of the gym that matters most! I think that we can all agree that the purpose of our bodies is not to show off on the treadmill or on the bench press machine, nor is it to flaunt a bare belly on Instagram. You might never be a size zero, and that is okay. The true purpose of our bodies is to use them! To explore the possibilities within ourselves and the world around us. To be strong, in all ways. To be confident to take action and opportunities because our strong, agile, healthy, and fit bodies can MOVE and BEND and LIFT and PUSH and PULL and LIVE.

Things change, and that's okay! Your body and your goals will and should change. In your twenties you might begin to work out to look great. By the time you hit twenty-five, the goal might shift as you transition from college life to working life; perhaps you'll be working out more for stress relief and balance. In your thirties, your goals might shift again—maybe your primary goal will be to work out to be healthy to have a baby. Your goals will change, and they should continue to do so into your forties and fifties and ideally onward. Your body will also go through changes in those years, and the only way to have control of as many of the variables we can is to have a consistent training routine, healthy clean eating, and an active lifestyle. As priorities, passions, and goals change, your dedication to yourself and your body should never change. Fitness should be a constant, a part of your life through all of it: the great, the challenging, the new, and even the stressful times.

Fitness should make you stronger. Physically, you deserve the right to feel capable and powerful and able-bodied. Compare yourself only to yourself and take full pride in your newfound abilities to move and experience your body pain-free and active. Mentally, your physical abilities—the milestones you will achieve and surpass in your workouts—will make you a stronger decision maker and overall a more confident person. You will soon see that you will not need anyone to build you up; your health and training will do that for you. Fitness should be the thing you go to when you feel a bit helpless or lost—your workouts will connect you with your innermost spirit, and all you have to do is take the time and put in the work. Trust me when I tell you that you will look forward to it and enjoy it. Eventually, your body will crave it. Your workouts will become the source from which you get your superpowers.

Be selfish. Being selfish for one hour or a half an hour a day will make you a far better, more clearheaded, less-stressed, happier, and more giving mother, daughter, coworker, wife, sister, friend, and even pet owner. By taking a small slice of the day for yourself and your personal development in your workouts, you will become a happier and more open-minded, energized, creative, relaxed version of yourself. You will have more energy to play with your kids, walk your dog, wrestle with your significant other, and get your work done. Never feel guilty about taking time for yourself—your loved ones deserve to have the best you around them . . . and the best you will be even better after a dedication to your mind, body, and spirit. Let your family members know this, and as you take the time each day, they will respect your process. Plus, you can serve as the best example to your family and friends. Your kids will copy you—don't you owe it to them to show them a healthy way?

Listen to your body, not your mind. Your mind is smart, and it will play tricks on you. Often your body can keep going and your mind says, "This is tough, this is hard . . . I want to stop." The moment you move past that thought and connect the mind and body together is the moment that you will master yourself. Your mind might say, "I am tired; I don't want to work out right now; this couch feels sooooo good!" Once you learn to cast those thoughts aside, you will stop having them. Instead of your mind speaking just for its instant gratification, it will begin to consult your body, and the two together will actually trigger a response that will have you counting down the hours between you and your next workout! During your workouts, you will learn to push forward instead of giving in and giving up—this type of mental and physical fortitude will translate into every single corner of your life. Soon you will see yourself as "that person," that girl who never gives up and never gives in and instead achieves.

Right now, today, and every day going forward: **celebrate your journey and forget about your destination.** Your journey is your new life. It is a life of movement, action, awareness, discovery, and effort without end. It's not a life for the lazy. It's the life of a traveler—the life of someone on a quest. If you do this correctly, you will want more and more challenges even past your initial goals. Just take everything day by day and enjoy it. Even the tough days—enjoy them.

Continue to challenge yourself, as you did in your first week. You have to continue to discover yourself, as you did in your second and third weeks.

Accept yourself. This might actually be the hardest task of all. Accept yourself! You *must* accept yourself. Most people fail because they want the world to unfold for them in a week or two, but that is simply not the case. It can't. It takes time. When people see changes in the first week or two they get excited. But by week four, too often I see people become discouraged because they can't accept themselves—they want change to come in an instant. You didn't gain all of your weight in four weeks. It took years to gain weight and lose mobility and strength. And now you want those years of poor habits to simply be wiped clean in four weeks. It's the wrong attitude, and this type of thinking leads to failure.

Don't worry! It doesn't mean that it will take you years to regain your shape, strength, and health. Luckily, in my experience, 30, 60, or 90 days sets you on a great path. But still, there is always a continued effort. Do not look at the end result. Envision your goals in steps, enjoy those steps, and keep on going. You must accept yourself first, and you must keep moving. Keep up the routine, the training, the eating, and the personal discipline.

That is the ultimate life change, to accept yourself and STILL keep going. That, and only that, will empower you to live the kind of life that will lock in your fitness forever. You can do this. You only have a little further to go.

The concepts I discuss are simple, and yet sometimes we ignore them. We say the words, "tomorrow" or "next week" or "on Monday! I will begin on Monday." Cast that aside too—excuses can go on forever, and soon a year will pass, then two. Do not cast yourself in a mold; human beings are too beautiful, and we have too much potential to remain the same and not evolve. Your job is to become a better version of yourself every single day. This will give you a level of satisfaction and fulfillment that very few other things can. I urge you to try. Every single person deserves to experience the feeling of being their best—physically, mentally, and spiritually.

In the end **I am here.** I want you to know that I am going through the same challenges you are every day. And together we will train, learn to eat clean, and tap into a better version of ourselves. Every time you do a workout, know that I am doing it too, and so are the thousands of women working out with Kettlebell

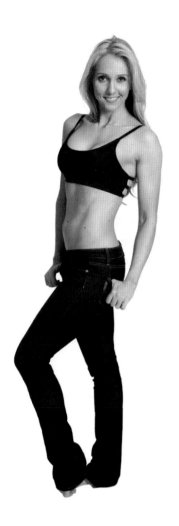

Kickboxing DVDs, or reading this book, or even doing the physical classes with me in New York City and in the countless other cities and countries that I visit. When you feel a bit lost for motivation, or even when you want to share an accomplishment or a thought, visit us on our social media and blog and share or just read and scroll through the posts and comments of other Kettlebell Kickboxers. Our Instagram account @KettlebellKickboxing has thousands of followers, and I post updates several times a day, including workout videos, step-by-steps, studio and success pictures, and recipes. Our Twitter @KBKickboxing shares the same content. Our Facebook page has updates and a wonderful community as well as the opportunity to ask questions. And our blog on kettlebellkickboxing.com has a wealth of information that follows every concept discussed in this book!

Join the community; it is full of like-minded individuals just like you. Use hashtags #KettlebellKickboxing and #KBBody so that we can find you.

INDEX OF MOVES

ABOUT THE AUTHOR

Dasha Libin Anderson has a master's degree in sports science and a variety of other training certifications including a specialty in performance enhancement and injury prevention (NASM-PES) with the National Academy of Sports Medicine, a speed and explosion specialty (NASE-SES) with the National Association of Speed and Explosion, and an MKC-2 ranking with Steve Maxwell. She holds instructor credentials in a variety of martial arts practices she has studied under her longtime instructor and husband, Dan Anderson. At their NYC studio, Anderson's Martial Arts Academy, she teaches sold-out Kettlebell Kickboxing classes. She spent over a decade developing the Kettlebell Kickboxing program, which is based on science and experience and is now accredited by the National Academy of Sports Medicine, National Strength and Conditioning Association, and American Council on Exercise. Dasha was named *NY1*'s New Yorker of the Week for her free women's self-defense program and was featured as *Black Belt*'s Twenty-First-Century Martial Artist. Dasha has been sponsored by Lululemon, Victoria's Secret Sport, and Athleta. She has worked with Nike and was the official trainer for the Miss New York USA and Miss Teen USA brands. She has worked on fitness features with *Self*, *Women's Health*, and *Shape* and has been written about in *Vanity Fair*, *Fitness*, and the *Wall Street Journal*. She lives in New York City.

**To find out more about Kettlebell Kickboxing and
to shop for DVDs including:**

Scorcher Series
Body Series
7-Day Lean Series
Scorcher Series 2.0

visit kettlebellkickboxing.com.